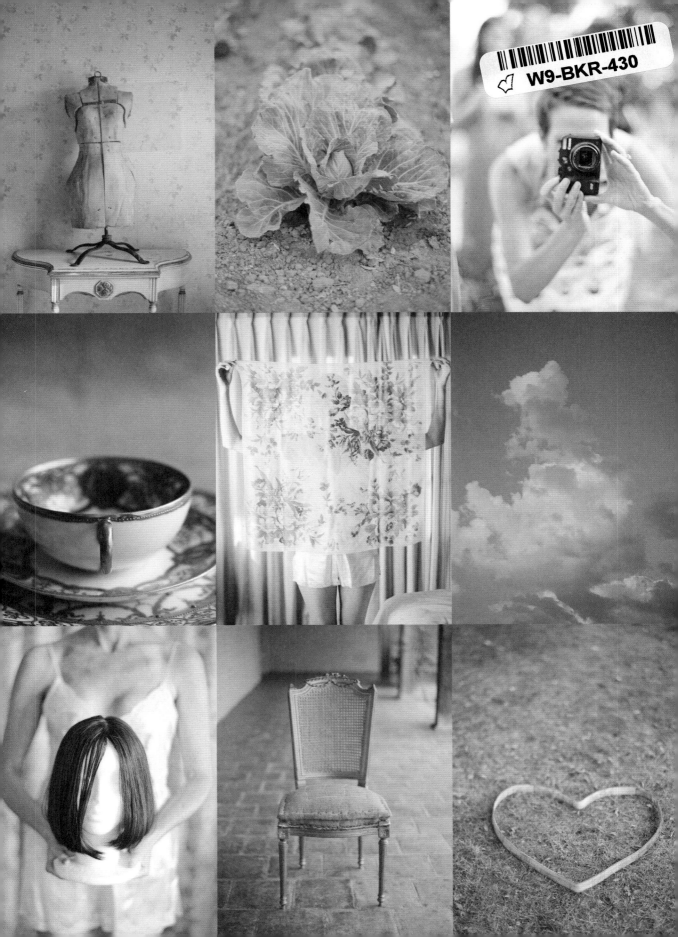

The Silver Lining

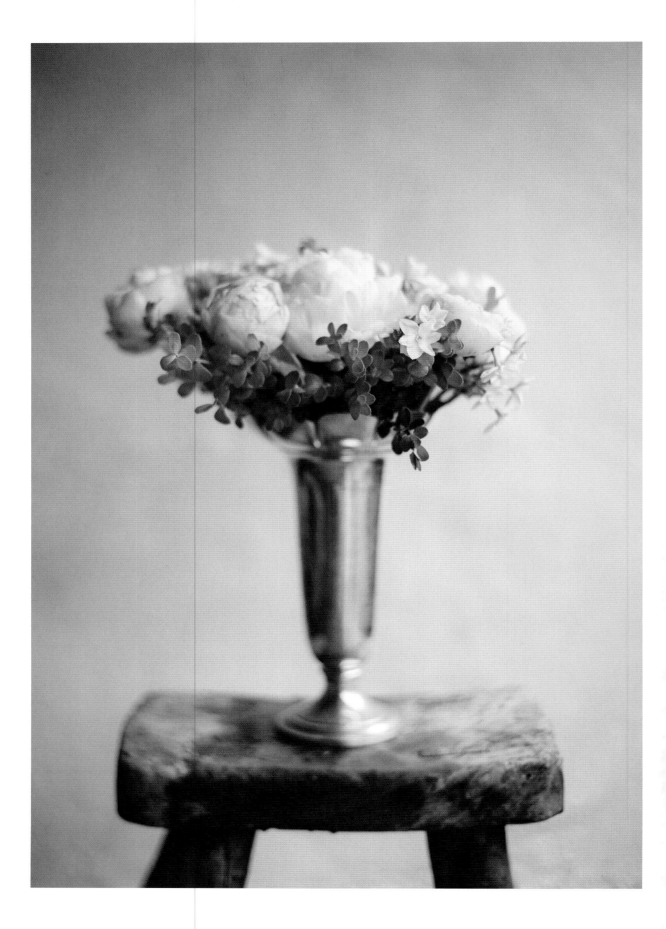

The Silver Lining

A SUPPORTIVE AND INSIGHTFUL GUIDE TO BREAST CANCER

HOLLYE JACOBS, RN, MS, MSW

PHOTOGRAPHS BY ELIZABETH MESSINA

ATRIA BOOKS

NEW YORK LONDON TORONTO SYDNEY NEW DELHI

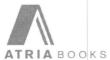

ATRIA BOOKS

A Division of Simon & Schuster, Inc.
1230 Avenue of the Americas
New York, NY 10020

This publication contains the opinions and ideas of its authors. It is intended to provide
helpful and informative material on the subjects addressed in the publication. It is sold with
the understanding that the authors and publisher are not engaged in rendering medical,
health, or any other kind of personal professional services in the book. The reader should
consult his or her medical, health, or other competent professional before adopting any
of the suggestions in this book or drawing inferences from it. The authors and publisher
specifically disclaim all responsibility for any liability, loss, or risk, personal or otherwise,
which is incurred as a consequence, directly or indirectly, of the use and application of any of
the contents in this book.

First Atria Books hardcover edition March 2014

ATRIA BOOKS and colophon are trademarks of Simon & Schuster, Inc.

For information about special discounts for bulk purchases, please contact
Simon & Schuster Special Sales at 1-866-506-1949 or business@simonandschuster.com.

The Simon & Schuster Speakers Bureau can bring authors to your live event.
For more information or to book an event contact the Simon & Schuster Speakers
Bureau at 1-866-248-3049 or visit our website at www.simonspeakers.com.

Interior design by Doug Turshen with David Huang
Jacket design by Doug Turshen with David Huang
Jacket art by Elizabeth Messina

Manufactured in China

10   9   8   7   6   5   4   3   2   1

Library of Congress Control Number: 2013010103

ISBN 978-1-4767-6350-7
ISBN 978-1-4767-4371-4 (pbk)
ISBN 978-1-4767-4372-1 (ebook)

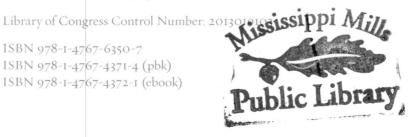

For my HOTY & children.
You are my ultimate Silver Linings.
—HOLLYE JACOBS

For my loving parents,
Josephine & Michael.
—ELIZABETH MESSINA

Behind
every cloud
is a
Silver Lining

—PROVERB

Contents

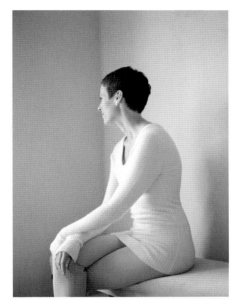

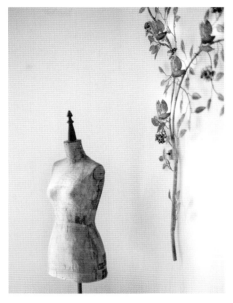

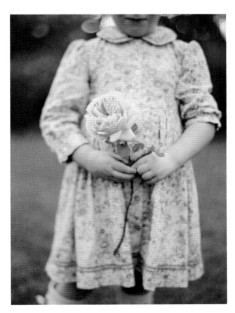

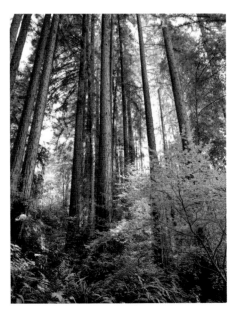

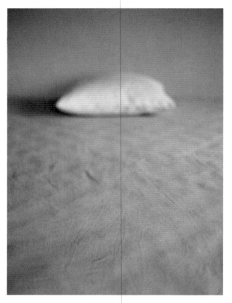

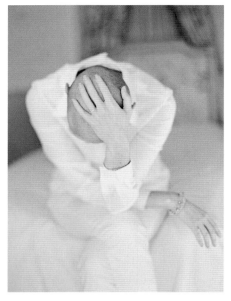

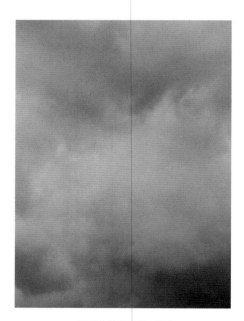

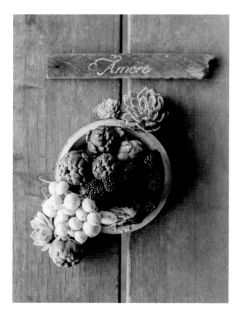

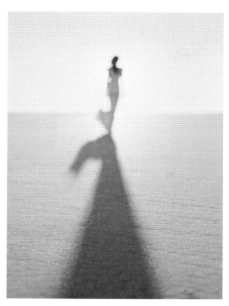

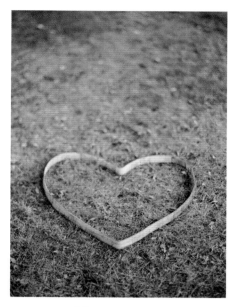

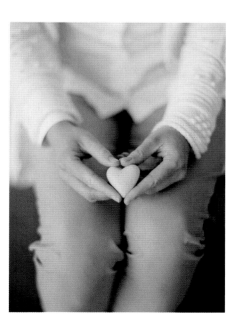

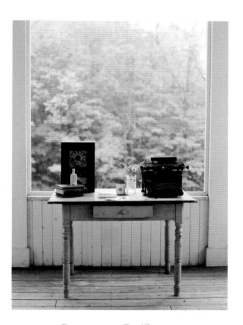

Introduction

As a happily married wife, mother, palliative care nurse, and social worker living in bucolic Santa Barbara, California, I was stunned by my breast cancer diagnosis (understatement of the century). I mean, really. I was a healthy, happy, vegan-eating, marathon-running thirty-nine-year-old with no family history of breast cancer.

As a bookworm, I first thought, "I need the perfect book to get me through this." What I needed was a lifeline, a guide and point of reference, a source of encouragement that was simultaneously honest and informative, practical and supportive, beautiful and serious, realistic and uplifting. No such book existed. So, I decided to write the book that I desperately sought, but could not find, after my breast cancer diagnosis. This book is for you.

The story is fundamentally my journey of self-discovery through illness, finding Silver Linings in life, and celebrating grace and positive thinking from the time of my breast cancer diagnosis through treatment, recovery, and ultimately the celebration of life after breast cancer.

Why Silver Linings? you ask. Well, I've always been a "half-full" kind of girl. It's easy to be half-full when life is good, when wondering what to make for dinner is the most pressing issue of the day. However, my half-fullness was first challenged in my professional life as a hospice nurse, caring for both dying adults and dying children, and then in my personal life when I became a cancer patient.

In my clinical practice as a hospice nurse, I vividly remember caring for a woman with breast cancer. She was in her late forties, with two young daughters. I remember playing on the floor of the living room of the hospital unit with the girls, feeling utterly helpless because I didn't know what to say or do with them. After all, I was in my late twenties. I wasn't yet a mother. And I hadn't been trained in talking with children.

Yet, somehow this woman—this dying woman—put the staff at ease by talking about all of the positive things in her life, the things that brought her joy, such as watching her children play, the smell of food cooking (even if she couldn't eat it), having a day without pain. She taught the staff—and, more important, her daughters—about resilience and finding Silver Linings and seeing the light—even a sliver—in the darkest circumstances.

Fast-forward to October 2010. When I heard the words "You have breast cancer," my first thought—literally my first thought—was: "This could be so much worse. My form of cancer is treatable."

As a nurse and social worker, I now found myself *in* the hospital bed. As a patient, I gained a whole new and unexpected conscious sensitivity to the physical and emotional aspects of being a patient, from becoming a human pincushion to contending with the common feelings of sadness, fear, and anxiety.

In fact, between my diagnosis and surgery, I felt lost and overwhelmed. I went through a period of internal struggle during which part of me was feeling like the lead character in *Life of Pi*: alone at sea with no clue where I was and a ginormous tiger in my boat.

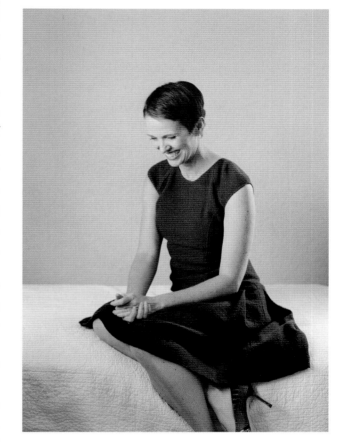

Before I allowed myself to be eaten by this tiger I gave myself a *Moonstruck* "snap out of it" moment and reminded myself of the woman for whom I cared in hospice. I remembered feeling so inspired by her resilience—her ability to cope with stress and adversity—in the face of overwhelming odds, that from the moment of my diagnosis, I consciously chose to look for the positive, the Silver Linings.

Now here's the thing about Silver Linings: unfortunately (!) they don't take away the pain, nausea, mouth sores, or constipation that can come with a cancer diagnosis and treatment, but they do provide balance, perspective, and hope.

When you have cancer, Silver Linings come in small and big packages. From watching a hummingbird outside my bedroom window (because I was too sick to stand), to enduring a side effect–filled treatment, to being cancer free (after enduring the longest and most painful year of my life), I know that Silver Linings are always present. All one has to do is look for them.

I realized that I had two choices about how I was going to handle my diagnosis: from a place of fear or from a place of optimism. I chose—and it was indeed a very active choice for me—optimism in the form of finding Silver Linings. There were many days when finding Silver Linings was a really, really hard choice. On one or two occasions I even doubted whether it was possible to find them. However, I did, because Silver Linings are always there.

This book evolved from my blog, *The Silver Pen*. I started writing the blog shortly after my diagnosis to keep my family and friends apprised of what was going on with me during my treatment. Prior to my diagnosis, as a nurse and a social worker, I had written a few academic papers and a couple of book chapters, but I had never written about myself. *Gulp.*

The truth is that I started writing so that I wouldn't have to talk with people and field the same well-meaning and lovingly intended but—for a patient—unbearable question of "How are you?" over and over again. How many times could I say, "I feel horrendous"?

I was thinking of my family as well. I didn't want them to be burdened with having to repeat stories over and over again. So if my husband wanted to get away from Cancerville (the name of our home for a year) and go out for the evening, when people asked how I was, he could say, "Read *The Silver Pen*. Hollye writes everyday."

So, *The Silver Pen* became my personal experience with cancer, written through the lens of my professional experience. An unexpected Silver Lining was that in a fairly short period of time, the blog went viral. What started as a way to communicate with family and friends became a source of information and—so I'm told—inspiration that gives a descriptive voice to the breast cancer experience.

This book, with its balance of substance, beauty, humor, and hope, artfully provides the opportunity to see the breast cancer experience from both sides of the bed, from the perspective of an experienced nurse and that of a close friend. Though I can't prepare you for everything that you may (or may not) experience during your treatment, what I can do is hold your hand and guide you through the process.

The photographic collaboration with Elizabeth was an unanticipated Silver Lining of my illness that began, as many wonderful things do, over a laugh and a cry. Shortly after my surgery, in a gesture of friendship, Elizabeth offered to photograph me. Her vision—literally and figuratively—was one of the brightest and most insightful lights in this dark period. When I looked in the mirror, the reflection that I saw was of the ravages of cancer. Elizabeth's gift of love, through her imagery, was to show my true reflection. She enabled me to see that I was still Me, full of light, love, and joy. I hope that this book, told through words and photography, will inspire, inform, and support you throughout your journey.

—Hollye Jacobs

The day that Hollye told me that she had breast cancer, I felt haunted with helplessness. I wanted to hug her, to bring her flowers. I wanted to do something, but nothing seemed quite right. I did not want to burden her with my fear and sadness. I also knew that I could not eliminate the intensity of the path that lay in front of her.

In thinking about what I could do for her, I reflected on moments in my life of extreme trauma and emotion, including the time when my oldest daughter was gravely ill as an infant. I remembered the profound intensity of being so aware of every moment and yet later not being able to remember much of that time. It was then that I realized that I wanted to give Hollye the gift of memory through photographs. Having images from her experience would enable her, should she ever wish, to reflect on and digest her journey.

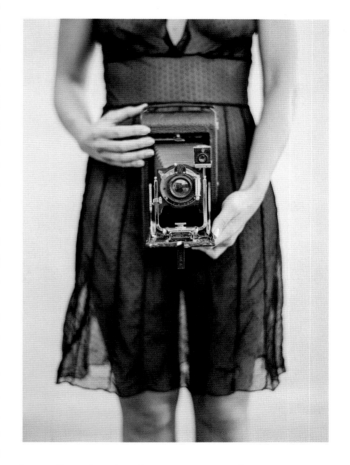

This was something that, as a photographer and her friend, I could do for and give to her. It was important to me to reflect Hollye's genuine beauty in the most unlikely of circumstances. During our time together, we shared a mutual bond of compassion and thoughtfulness mixed with genuine tenderness and robust humor.

Life for all of us is fraught with challenges, pain, and loss. There is nothing beautiful about cancer. There is, however, profound beauty in the human experience. I hoped that Hollye would be able to see herself not just as a cancer patient but also as a woman, full of grace and beauty.

These photographs were originally created as a personal gift from one friend to another. It wasn't until more than a year after I began photographing Hollye's journey that we began to envision them as part of a book. Now, these personal photographs are here, in *The Silver Lining,* as a gift for all. My hope is that the softness and beauty found in some unlikely moments will help you or someone you love embrace the grace that is within us all, even in the most unimaginable circumstances.

—Elizabeth Messina

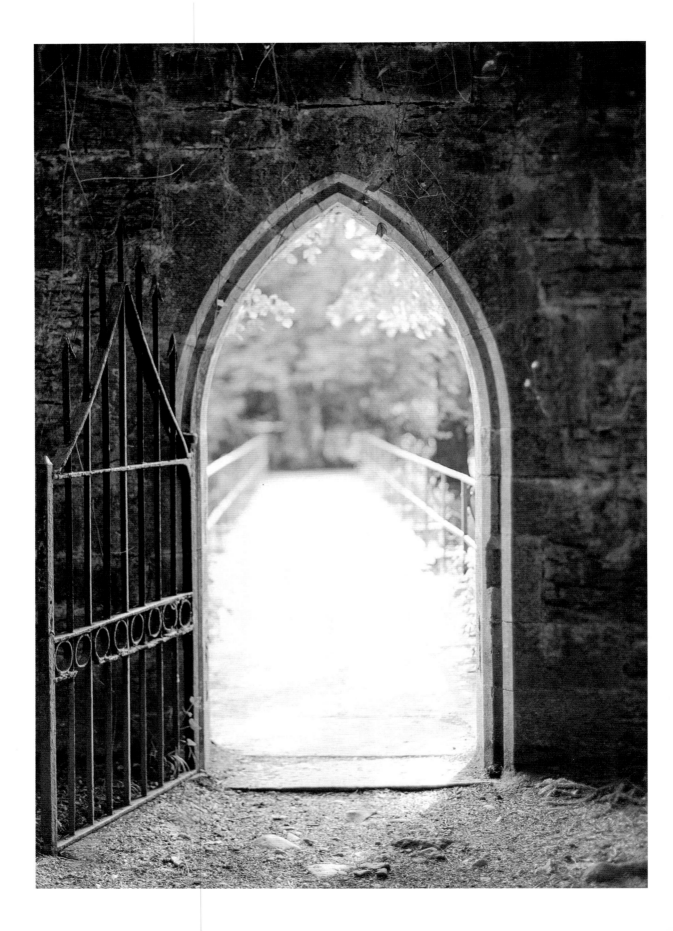

How to Use This Book

The Silver Lining is the book that I wish I'd had during my experience with breast cancer; therefore, I have intentionally written and organized it in the way that I would have preferred to read it. Because everyone diagnosed with breast cancer has a different course of therapy, I have separated each potential treatment into individual chapters, including surgery ("Lost & Found"), chemotherapy ("Chemo Sobby"), and radiation ("Radiation Cloud"). Since talking with children, nutrition, recovery, and life after breast cancer are unique and separate aspects of having the disease, I've given each topic its own chapter.

Each chapter is subdivided into three sections: Memoir, The Silver Lining, and Practical Matters. The first section is the chronicle of my experience, including the highs, the lows, and everything in between. When you feel like laughing, please do. There are some ridiculous experiences that still make me laugh when I think about them. Truth be told, you may need a tissue or two as well. I know that I did.

Within the memoir section, I offer you "Lifelines." These are the suggestions for you to learn from my experiences, both personal as well as professional, and even better yet, prevent some of the calamities (oh yes, calamities) that I faced.

The second section of each chapter is quite possibly my favorite. It is called "The Silver Lining." Because Silver Linings buoyed me throughout my entire experience, it is important to me to share my poignant sources of hope and inspiration with you, with high hopes that they also provide balance, perspective, and inspiration to support this exceptionally lumpy (pun intended) breast cancer road.

The third section of each chapter is called "Practical Matters." This title is specifically named because from the time of a diagnosis through treatment and beyond, the *practical* does indeed *matter*. The content in "Practical Matters" pertains to those necessary things, from information to action steps that are important to know during every phase of treatment and recovery. I wanted to make it as easy as possible to access helpful information. For example, the night before surgery, you can go to this section and get a list of what to take to the hospital or, before a doctor's appointment, you can readily access a list of questions to ask.

Now, you may be wondering: What's up with these photos? Well, I remember laying in my bed as a bald skeleton, wishing that I had a book on my nightstand that was simultaneously beautiful and helpful, inviting and supportive. Elizabeth and I have carefully and thoughtfully placed the photographs in this book to help guide, uplift, inform, and encourage you through the process. We believe that these beautiful images will bring peace and comfort on days that you don't have the energy to read or they will help you take a nice deep breath on a hard day. Our intention is not to make the breast cancer experience beautiful, but rather to add some beauty to the experience.

—Hollye Jacobs, RN, MS, MSW

CHAPTER I

An Interruption
The Breast Cancer Diagnosis

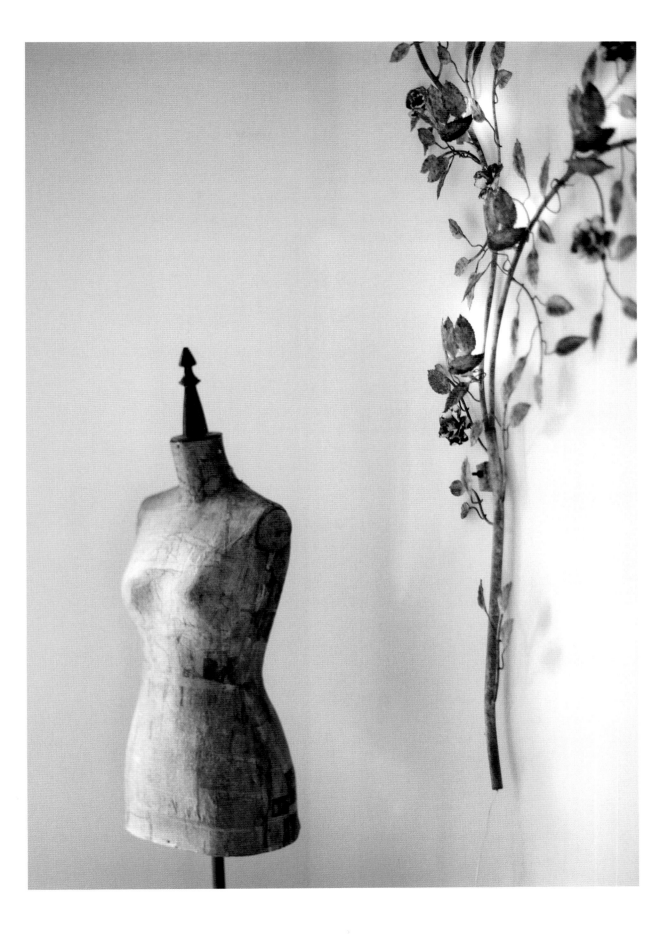

I'm fortunate to have had a myriad of professional experiences in my life, all seemingly disparate—until now. I started working for Ralph Lauren in Indiana at the age of sixteen because I loved fashion and desired some financial autonomy. Yes, my control issues started at a young age!

I went on to attend Saint Mary's College at Notre Dame, where I studied political science and history. My college experience was extraordinary. A liberal arts education taught me how to think, learn, write, and communicate, all foundational and fundamental skills for doing anything in life. Even though I adored my majors, I had a secret longing to be a nurse. However, I was raised hearing "You're not good at math and science." As children are apt to do, I believed what I was told and constrained my education to the humanities.

After graduation, I worked in retail at the Ralph Lauren store in Chicago for a number of years, selling clothes and hosting parties. The day that a woman screeched at me over an issue with a forty-nine-dollar shirt, I decided that I needed to add balance and perspective to my life and began pursuing my closeted dream of being a nurse. Guess what? As it turns out, I *am* good at math and science, earning an A+ in organic chemistry and going on to graduate—with honors—from Loyola University Chicago's accelerated bachelor's degree in nursing.

My first job in nursing was as a cardiovascular intensive care unit (ICU) nurse in the level III trauma center at Loyola University Chicago on the night shift. Sleep has always been very important to me. This was the first time in my life that I had to stay awake *all* night. To describe it as challenging is an understatement. I'll never forget being so tired one day when I came home (at seven thirty in the morning after a twelve-hour shift) that when I took my dog out for his morning constitutional, I put my mail in the trash can and his poop in the mailbox. Oh yes, I did. And I'm still mortified about it!

In my job as an ICU nurse, my work was excruciatingly intense and filled with extraordinary amounts of blood, guts, and death. Many people who intentionally spend their entire careers on the night shift do so either because it is better for their family-work balance or because generally they don't like people and don't like for their patients to be awake. I'm afraid that I worked with too many people who didn't like for their patients to be awake.

I'll never forget one of my colleagues, "Nurse Ratched," who asked, "Why in heaven's name do you smile so much? What is there to be happy about?" Startled, I responded, "I'm just a happy person. I happen to think that there are a lot of things to be happy about, beginning with the fact that I'm not one of the patients in these

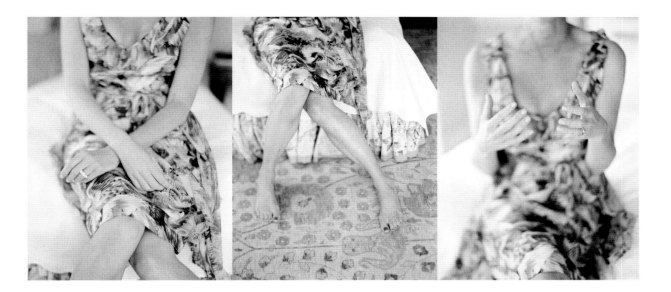

beds." Her response—you're never going to believe it—was, "If I do one thing while you're here—and you're not going to be here for very long—I'm going to wipe that smile off your face." You know what I did? I laughed. Now, it was a terrified, shriek-filled, crazy laugh, but she never spoke to me like that again (perhaps because she thought I was nuts).

As the nurse in charge of delegating patient care, Nurse Ratched always assigned me to care for the patients who were dying. I think that this was her attempt to wipe the smile off my face; however, there was a great Silver Lining to those assignments because it took me to my vocation, working in the field of hospice. I believe that there is no greater gift or honor in the world than to be present with someone at the beginning of life or at the end of life. It's not to say that end-of-life care is easy or that it is not sad. Many times, the work is heartbreaking. However, for whatever reason, in the middle of the night in the ICU, I found my calling.

Speaking of calling, it was during this period that I met my husband. Ours was not a love-at-first-sight kind of story, but we had an immediate and strong connection. There were some, well, constraining factors that put up roadblocks to the potential for romance. Where to start? Well, he was in the middle of a divorce, raising three boys, running an important company as well as a foundation, *and* he happened to be Jewish (I was raised Catholic). Oh and he was twenty years older. The fact that I had two jobs, was in graduate school, and had a happy dating life were additional constraints to a budding la-di-da, Cupid-instigated romance.

When interesting, unique, or even rotten experiences happen to me, I'm not one to ask "Why?" Instead, I'm apt to wonder, "What is the purpose of this experience? What am I supposed to learn from it? Where is the growth opportunity?"

So, in meeting my husband-to-be, whom I didn't know was my husband-to-be, I put one and one together and found that it made eleven. I found out that we shared a passion for fun, food, laughter, travel, and, most important, child advocacy. We also shared a passion for making the world a better place. I assumed that these shared passions were the explanation for our meeting.

During the course of the next year, we developed a beautiful friendship. We talked multiple times a day (this was pre-email, Facebook, Instagram, Twitter, text, and IM'ing, so we had an old-fashioned, talk-on-the-phone kind of friendship) and saw each other several days per week. He was the first person I talked with when I woke up in the morning and the last person I talked with before going to sleep. We grew closer and closer until one day the clouds parted and the Silver Linings (though I didn't identify them by name yet) appeared, as if saying, "Helloooooooooo? Here he is, right in front of you. Yes, you are both ready. It's time . . ."

And, just like that, we transitioned from a deep and meaningful friendship to an exciting and powerful romantic relationship. It was a huge leap of faith because I treasured our friendship; however, my intuition said, "Yes. This is right."

In the meantime, professionally, it was at the suggestion of my now boyfriend and future husband that I made the leap from the ICU to the field of hospice and palliative care, working in the light of day, I might add.

Please allow me to tell you a little bit about hospice. It is a philosophy and type of care that focuses on providing relief of a person's physical, emotional, spiritual, or social symptoms at the end of life. An interdisciplinary team of health care providers—made up of nurses, physicians, social workers, chaplains, volunteers, music therapists, and other complementary practitioners—deliver hospice care. The best part of this care is the interdisciplinary approach because it means that a team of people brings particular expertise to the situation with the sole (or is it soul?) purpose of meeting any and all needs of patients and their families.

In moving to this field full-time, I had an incredibly steep and inspirational learning curve. One minute I wanted to throw up because I was so nervous about caring for people who were actually *dying,* and the next minute I felt like I was doing the work that I was born to do.

During this period, as a young, vibrant, and ambitious nurse, I was presented with the most real of life's lessons. I came to the realization that death is not just for the old, the weary, and the infirm. Quite the contrary, death does not discriminate. We have all heard the tragic stories about random and senseless death and say, "Wow.

LIFELINE

Whether in health or in love, trust your intuition. It will point you in the right direction, always & in all ways.

That's awful. That's terrible." However, caring for a person in this circumstance is a Totally Different Deal.

Caring for a twenty-nine-year-old graduate student who was six months shy of a graduation that she would never attend was chilling. Caring for the forty-two-year-old father of two young children and knowing he would never see their weddings was devastating. Caring for the thirty-three-year-old marathon runner who would never run another race was stunning.

Caring for the adolescent boy who would not graduate from high school was haunting. What on earth was a teenager doing on our adult unit—as a *patient?*—you wonder. Heaven knows I did! His clinical and socioeconomic circumstances were so challenging that we were the only hospice program in Chicago that would take him. I felt completely and totally incompetent. Holy moly. However, our team, led by an indomitable social worker, pulled together and cared for this young boy and his family. It was heart wrenching, but as his mother told us later, we provided him and his family with a peaceful, pain-free death.

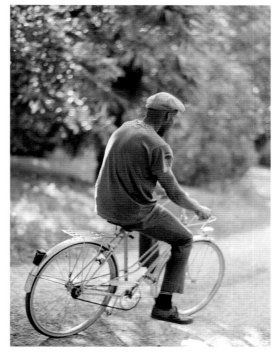

Because I wanted to be prepared if I was ever in the position of caring for another child, I did everything I could possibly do to educate myself so that I would feel fully competent and capable to do this work, including hands-on clinical training and hours on end in the library (yes, I know I'm dating myself!). I also proceeded to obtain graduate degrees in bioethics, child development, and social work. As it turned out, I came to the surprising realization that I had the capacity to care for dying children and their families. I have no clue how it happened, but I found myself drawn to pediatric hospice.

As a pediatric hospice nurse, I did both clinical work with families and also taught. Teaching and learning are two of the great loves of my life. Growing—intellectually, emotionally, and spiritually—is such a gift. Because I wanted all of the children who needed hospice services to receive them, I felt compelled to teach students and clinicians how to care for children and their families facing the end of life. So, I taught a class to medical students at the University of Chicago. I also ran the City of Hope End-of-Life Nursing Education Consortium (ELNEC) Pediatric Palliative Care program. This is a train-the-trainer course that teaches nurses and other health care professionals how to do hospice and palliative care.

Being one hundred percent present with a person who is dying gave me a perspective on life that transformed my soul. It also inspired me. In caring for people who were dying I grew emotionally, socially, intellectually, and spiritually. There was no way I could not. In my late twenties, I learned that life can turn on a dime. This realization inspired me to live each day to the fullest, as presently as I could possibly be. Little did I know—how could I?—that this realization would become personal.

In the meantime, my personal life proceeded on a beautiful path, though not without extraordinary challenges. My husband-to-be and I forged an incredible partnership based on mutual trust and a commitment to the no-matter-what kind of love. The path to our marriage was laden with personal toxicity and pain the likes of which I would never wish on anyone. However, against all odds, we found peace, harmony, love, and joy.

What I didn't know at the time was that both my personal relationship with my husband and my professional life as a nurse were preparing me for the biggest and most demanding experience of my life. Every bit of my half-fullness was on the precipice of being challenged on a grand scale. It's easy to be half-full when things proceed swimmingly in life. It's when things fall apart, when the clouds roll in, that we have the opportunity to see the Silver Linings in life and in people.

THE PAIN

December 18 is a terrible date for a birthday. A week before Christmas? C'mon. I can't count how many times I've heard "This is a combination birthday/Christmas gift." Really? Cue the annual pity party.

My 2010 birthday was going to be different, I promised myself. After all, it was my fortieth. I'm the only person I know who was truly excited about turning the big 4-0. Perhaps it was the fact that I have been a hospice nurse for many years and I've seen way too many people not live to see their fortieth birthday. The "gift" cliché is no cliché to me.

After thirty-nine years of never having had a real birthday party (no, not even as a child), I didn't feel the need to start with number forty. Instead, my husband and I decided to celebrate this milestone with a magnificent trip to New Zealand. Dreamy, right?

I had to keep the dream just that, a dream, because on September 28, 2010, three months shy of that exciting birthday, I was awakened by a sharp, shooting pain in my right breast. I felt like I was being stabbed with an ice pick.

I happen to be a person who can sleep standing up, with the lights on and a live band playing (yes, this has actually happened). So, to be awakened was a rare

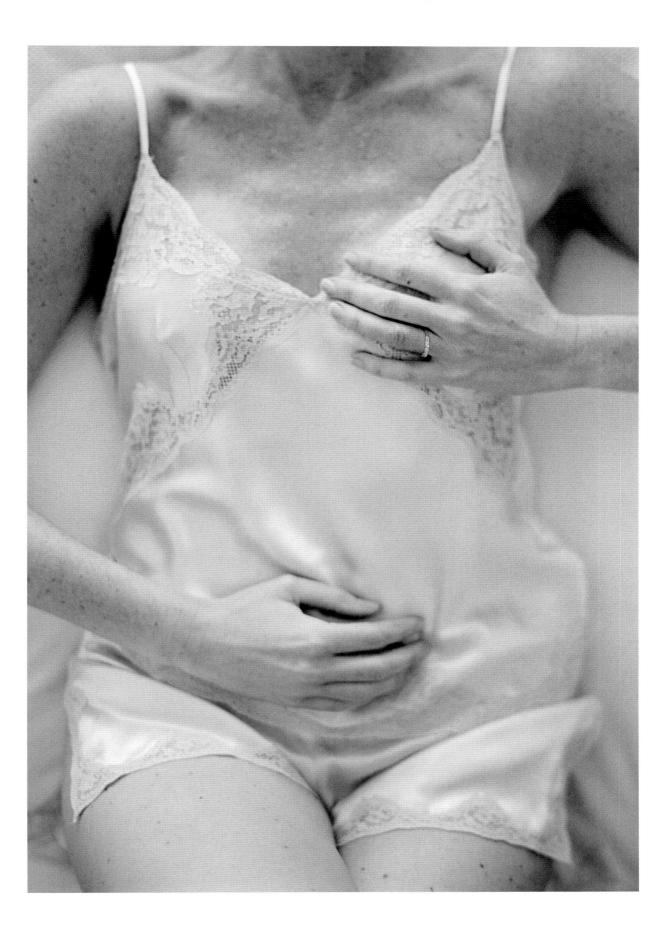

occurrence for me. Touching the phantom puncture wound, I immediately felt a lump in my right breast and thought, "What on *earth* is this?"

I don't consider myself an alarmist and promptly went back to sleep. Two days later, the exact same thing happened. I now thought, this *isn't* right. However, reminding myself that I am not an alarmist, I erroneously told myself that the lump was a cyst (a fluid-filled sac) that is common in women my age and was a result of drinking coffee, a new and unfortunate habit to which I had succumbed as a result of omnipresent fatigue. These cysts are usually harmless and can be painful. After it happened the second time, I told my husband.

Any potential worries were assuaged because, as a nurse, I assured myself and my now worried husband that breast cancer usually doesn't hurt ("usually" turned out to be the operative word). Furthermore, just a month previously, I had had a full checkup (including a breast exam!) with my internist, who deemed me to be in perfect health.

Despite my best efforts, worries seemed to keep creeping onto our radar. I already had a checkup scheduled with a new gynecologist the following week. Because we had just moved to Santa Barbara, one of the many things on my to-do list was to schedule checkups with new doctors. I assured myself that this pesky pain issue would be resolved then.

My overly concerned husband was not happy about delaying the appointment a week. "Why wait?" he asked. "Because, this week I have a business trip to Chicago and there is nothing to be concerned about," I said. "Why is he so antsy?" I wondered.

A week and three more middle-of-the-night pain awakenings later, I found myself at my gynecologist's office, where I (erroneously) assumed that she would tell me that the cyst was a result of overly ambitious coffee consumption and to cut out the caffeine. I had a full checkup, including blood work and all of the other unmentionable components of a gynecologic exam. I pointed out the prominently palpable (meaning that I could feel it) lump in my right breast.

My new doctor assured me that the lump was probably nothing. In all likelihood, it was a fluid-filled cyst, she said. Aha, just as I thought! There was a chance, however, that it could be a fibroadenoma, a benign solid tumor that is common in women in their twenties and thirties.

> **LIFELINE**
>
> *I've always been a big believer in regular checkups, even when you're healthy. What is the downside in having someone say "You're healthy!"? One of the upsides to having a regular doctor is that you have an established history from which you can draw if you, ahem, need to.*

To be sure that it was not a tumor, she wanted me to have a diagnostic mammogram and handheld ultrasound as soon as possible. ASAP? "Well," I wondered, "if she thinks it's 'nothing,' then why am I being rushed into these tests?" I kept waiting for her to tell me to stop drinking coffee.

Prior to leaving, I explained to her that I am a person who responds well to information, whether it is good or bad. Therefore, I asked her pointedly whether she thought I had breast cancer. "Absolutely not," she said. *Phew.*

That afternoon, I called the two places in Santa Barbara that do mammograms and handheld ultrasounds. The first available appointment at both locations was a minimum of three weeks away. Three weeks?!? However, one of the two said, "If you walk in promptly at eight thirty tomorrow morning, you will be the first person seen." A walk-in is something that I usually associate with nail appointments, not with mammogram and ultrasound appointments, but I had the ASAP comment looming in my mind. I told the receptionist that I would be there first thing the next morning.

In the meantime, my husband was packing for a couples trip to Israel, beginning the day before the "scheduled" walk-in appointment, though he was leaving without his half of said couple. This couples trip had been planned nearly a year in advance. At the onset of the planning, though I knew it would be an absolutely incredible, over-the-top trip, every ounce of my intuition told me that I was not supposed to be a part of it. Why? I had no idea.

Initially, my husband thought I was being ridiculous. For several months, we went back and forth about whether I would go. My wonderful, one-in-a-million husband rarely asks me for anything, so, at one point, I gave in to his rare request and signed up for five days, which equaled less than half of the trip. Who in her right mind goes to Israel from California for five days? you ask. A devoted Catholic wife!

Lo and behold, the day after I agreed to go, our travel agent called to say that the nonstop flight we were on was canceled and not replaced with any other viable option. Okay, if that wasn't a sign, I didn't know what was! After the inexplicable flight cancellation, my husband acquiesced and relieved me from any pressure whatsoever to attend. Because this trip was important to him, however, I supported his participation (even though I had an inkling that he, too, was not supposed to go).

Leaving the house for the airport, my husband said, "If you need a biopsy, wait until I get back." Really? *Ugh.*

THE TESTS

On the Thursday morning of my mammogram and handheld-ultrasound appointments, I drove myself to the radiology center. Inviting someone to come with me did not enter my realm of thinking. Why would it? Considering the conversation with my doctor, I had nothing to worry about.

After hearing horror mammogram stories about breasts being practically ripped off and smooshed (a more descriptive rather than clinical word) into a vise and then crushed, I must say that my mammogram experience was easy-peasy. My technician was incredibly kind and gentle. The only thing that teed me off a bit was when she said, "My best friend had breast cancer and she hiked during her chemo." Yes, she actually said this (&%@$✚#)!

Next up: handheld ultrasound. A handheld ultrasound uses wandlike devices that emit sound waves to identify abnormalities, lumps, and cysts. A breast ultrasound is typically recommended either when (in my case) a mass is palpable by hand or when a screening mammogram has shown something suspicious. It is used to determine if the abnormality is solid (such as a benign fibroadenoma or cancer) or fluid-filled (such as a benign cyst).

I was escorted in my ridiculously unchic gown to a quiet, dark room where, upon lying on the table with a warm blanket, I thought, "Wow. What a great place for an N-A-P!" The technician proceeded to have me raise my right arm over my head while she squirted a gel on my lumpy right breast. After, she gently guided a wand over my breast tissue to produce images on a nearby screen. It looked and felt much like a pregnancy ultrasound, with the absence of a beating heart and feelings of joy. Unfortunately, my nap was curtailed by the fact that the technician was chatty-chatty-chatty. She was so nice, though, that I couldn't be grumpy with her. I just closed my eyes, let her work and talk, and did little in the way of responding. After about ten minutes, she stopped talking. She instantly went from incessant chatter to radio silence. This, I knew, was a bad sign.

However, I took her silence as an opportunity to catch a little shut-eye. At one point, she asked me to stay in the room because she wanted to ask the radiologist whether he wanted a few more images. *Gulp.* "Do I have something to be worried about?" I wondered. "Impossible," I thought. Five minutes later, the technician returned and proceeded to squirt more gel on my lumpy right breast and then my left breast (for good measure?) to obtain more images.

When she finished, she asked me to put my clothes on and wait in the reception area. I asked when I would get the results (hoping for twenty-four hours). She told me that the radiologist would see me before I left. *Gulp.* Another bad sign.

When I was finally called into the radiologist's office, the images of my breasts were on four large monitors. He said, "I understand that you are a nurse."

"Yes," I said.

"Then, I assume that I can talk with you more directly than I could someone else," he said.

"Sure," I said. I looked down at my hands and saw that they were shaking. I felt as if I were about to be in a car crash, where everything happens before you know it but feels like slow motion.

"You have four tumors in your right breast and three in your left breast," he said. "We need to do a biopsy today and an MRI as soon as possible. Here are the images. You can see right here . . ." I instantly felt my heart race and my mind numb. I reminded myself to breathe, just breathe.

As a nurse, I know that patients forget virtually everything that comes after hearing the dreaded words "You have a tumor." So instinctively I knew that I would forget what I was about to hear and needed to write down as much as I possibly could.

The radiologist proceeded to introduce me to my lesions (i.e., tumors). I wondered: How did they get there so fast? And why are they so *big*? Just one month ago a doctor told me that I was a completely healthy thirty-nine-year-old woman without an inkling of anything going on anywhere, and now a radiologist was referring to my *tumors*? Was this *really* happening?

The radiologist then asked whether I was available for a biopsy that afternoon at three o'clock. I told him that of course I would be available. He told me that I should probably bring a friend with me. *Really? Ya think?*

By this time, after thirty-six hours of traveling, my husband had just landed in Israel and was on his way to dinner. Instead of calling him first, I called my best friend, whose nickname is LiFT (because of her initials, but little did I know how literal this nickname would become). LiFT had gone through the exact same thing a year and a half prior. No kidding. We went to nursing school together. We think the exact same way. I was with her at her diagnosis appointment, during her surgery, and at her last chemo treatment. After dropping a few naughty words, she said, "This is really awful news, and it's going to be a full year of sucky treatment, but at least We. Know. How. To. Do. This."

My first question to LiFT was, "When do I tell my husband?" He had just landed—in *Israel*—for goodness' sake. I figured that nothing was really going to happen in the next five days, so it would be better to wait until he got home to tell him. After all, I presumed that this was probably the last worry-free trip that he was going to take for a long, long time.

Ironically, LiFT's husband was on a weekend-long fishing trip when she received her diagnosis. At the time, we talked through the exact same "Do I tell him or do I let him enjoy his trip?" dilemma. As a gesture of thoughtful consideration, she decided to wait to tell him when he got home on Sunday night. After all, nothing would happen over the weekend. LiFT told me that she felt like this was the only wrong decision that she'd made throughout her entire treatment and that my husband needed to get his fanny on a plane and come home.

Driving down the 101 highway (which happened to be a construction zone), I made the call to my husband. Not the best timing for the delivery of the news, by the way. In fact, I'm so grateful that I didn't crash my car into one of the barriers. I managed to say, "I have breast cancer" before bursting into tears. "I'm coming home" is all I remember him saying.

The next call was to my internist to talk through the events of the morning, which were now moving at lightning speed. Fortunately, I had the wherewithal to realize that I couldn't see the forest from the trees and needed some levelheaded, clear, clinical thinking.

His first response was, "Whoa. Whoa. Whoa. Slow down. This is ridiculous. Things are moving way too fast. I'm sure this is nothing, but the first thing you need to do is an MRI. If you do a biopsy first, then the MRI results can be skewed."

He explained that if the person doing the biopsy has to poke around—and it does happen—to get the tissue sample, then it can cause bruising. That bruising has the potential to look like another tumor on the MRI. He went on to say, "You need an MRI first and then you may or may not need a biopsy. A breast surgeon needs to oversee everything."

After talking with my internist, I breathed a lung-emptying sigh of relief. *Finally,* I thought, someone who is *not* an alarmist. He said, "I'll call

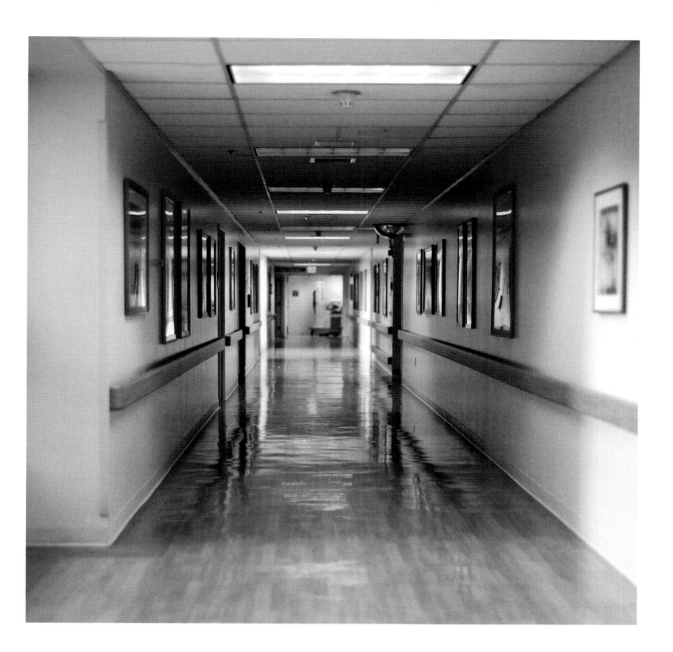

you back in five minutes." Precisely five minutes later he called, just like he said he would, and said, "Can you be downtown in fifteen minutes to meet with a surgeon?" Absolutely.

Back on the 101 highway, I felt much more cool, calm, and collected. After all, I was on my way to see a surgeon who would certainly tell me that this whole situation was just one big misunderstanding. Fifteen minutes later, I arrived at the surgeon's office and was promptly escorted into an exam room where my morning mammogram and ultrasound images were already up on the screen. "How'd they get there so fast?" I wondered. Impressive. The surgeon greeted me with a warm and calming smile and firm handshake. I felt instantly comfortable with her. She asked whether she could do a breast exam. After whipping my shirt off for the third stranger of the day, I hopped up on the table.

When she was finished with the breast exam, she said that she was "worried." She agreed that both an MRI and biopsy were in order. She gave me three options:

- Keep the three o'clock biopsy appointment with the radiologist.
- Get an MRI first and then have a biopsy (as recommended by my internist).
- Do the biopsy now, on the spot, and then send me for an MRI.

She assured me that if she did the biopsy, there would be no problem in doing an MRI afterward. That was code language for "Because of my surgical experience I won't miss the tumor. There will be no bruising that will skew MRI results." I trusted her surgeon's hands and said, "Let's do this. Now."

At this point, my exhausted and worried husband was en route home after spending a mere six hours in Israel. I had no clue where in the world he was. All I knew was that he was unreachable and that I couldn't wait until he got home to do the biopsy, as he had requested. I hoped that he would understand.

After I called to cancel the appointment at the radiology center, the surgeon proceeded to tell me that in the right breast she would do a fine-needle aspiration (FNA) of one of the tumors that was not palpable. After, she would do a large-core biopsy of the other, larger palpable lesion (the one that woke me up). The locations of the tumors were described in terms of a clock: the smaller tumor requiring the FNA was at one o'clock and the big momma was at nine o'clock. I don't think that a.m. or p.m. really matters, in case you were wondering.

As a nurse, I was fascinated with the process of both doing and watching a biopsy, especially *on* me. For the record, I do acknowledge how strange and twisted that is to say. I told her that I was a big advocate of pain management and to "go big" on the Lidocaine.

So, without pain, I watched as this skilled,

gentle, and thorough surgeon did biopsies on two of the lesions in my right breast.

The entire procedure took about fifteen minutes. When she was finished, as she was putting a Band-Aid on the biopsy sites, I asked her what she thought. She said, "Although I can't say for sure until I have the pathology report, I will say that I am very, very worried." As I was dressing, she gave me postprocedure instructions: "Call me if you have a fever over 101 degrees Fahrenheit, pain that is not relieved by over-the-counter pain medicine, swelling that does not go away, and/or continued bleeding."

My surgeon was eager for me to do the MRI that afternoon and was able to squeeze me in. I had never had a surgeon before. However, after someone sticks a whopper of a needle in your breast, you can then use a possessive description of him or her. She was now "my" surgeon.

The two of us had a conversation about the requested MRI. In reality, it was less dialogue and more my pleading and bargaining effort to do anything other than an MRI. A past experience with a closed MRI was forever embedded in my memory. Since I couldn't negotiate my way out of the exam, I told the surgeon that getting me into an itty-bitty claustrophobic tube was going to require *a lot* of mind-numbing medication. She pulled out her prescription pad and wrote an order for Valium.

In the meantime, this amazing surgeon told me that she didn't typically work on Fridays, but that she wanted to come in to discuss the preliminary test results (comprehensive pathology results would take several days). I told her that as a hospice and palliative care nurse, I had been in her chair—delivering bad news—and wanted to know ahead of time what she was going to tell me. All she said was, "I'm very, very worried." Enough said. I literally had to remind myself to keep breathing.

So, I called a local girlfriend (finally!) and, in order to ask her to escort my Valium-laden head to my MRI exam, I had to break the news.

When she didn't hesitate at my request and told me that she would meet me at my house in twenty minutes and drive me straight to the exam, I realized just how nice it was to no longer be doing this thing physically alone. In the meantime,

I stopped by the pharmacy to pick up the Valium. Just having the Valium in my possession helped me relax. Because of my claustrophobia, I was truly more stressed about the MRI than I was about my impending diagnosis.

LIFELINE

Take a friend or family member with you to any follow-up appointments. While you may be inclined to take your BFF, it is more important to take a person who you know will be cool as a cucumber to collect information & be a support to you!

As soon as we got in the car, I took the pill. My opiate naïveté (i.e., I am not in the habit of taking drugs) combined with the fact that I forgot to eat that day (a shocking occurrence in and of itself!) meant the Valium took effect almost immediately. As we were driving to the exam, my surgeon called and asked, "Have you taken the Valium yet?"

"Ohhhhhh, yesssssss," I said.

"Oh no," she said, "the MRI machine just broke."

"Toooooo baaaaaad," I dribbled.

"It is too bad because everything was going so well today."

"Foooooor whoooooom was it going well?" I asked my dear surgeon.

At least we both were able to laugh at that seriously laughable line. My surgeon rescheduled the MRI for the next morning at seven o'clock at a different location. With my Valium buzz still firmly in place, my girlfriend and I decided to run some plain old errands. After all, not everyone's world was rocked today, and errands still needed to be run. It was actually a gift for us to have time to process the events of the day.

It was at this point in the experience (perhaps because of the Valium) when I began recognizing and even naming all of the good things that were happening in the midst of this ridiculously overwhelming, life-altering situation:

- Being able to walk into the mammogram and ultrasound test.
- Having a responsive internist who helped me navigate the process.
- Meeting a competent and calming breast surgeon.
- Having steadfast, experienced, levelheaded girlfriends to help me through the process.

This was the moment when I began identifying Silver Linings. After all, these were true Silver Linings in a very dark and stormy day. They helped me maintain both perspective and a positive, hopeful attitude.

THE DIAGNOSIS

Fast-forward to six forty-five Friday morning, twenty-two hours after my mammogram, ultrasound, and biopsy tests. My girlfriend picked me up to drive me to the MRI appointment. My husband was still flying home. Having taken another Valium, I was completely relaaaaaaaxed. When I arrived, the woman at the desk said that they were going to have to wait to do the MRI because they didn't have the official doctor's order. *Reaaaaaaaallly?* I think that she saw the devastated look on my face and said, "I know, it's coming. Let's get you in, sweetie." Here was another Silver Lining!

Not only did I survive the MRI but I fell asleep in it! The technician had to wake me up. At this point I began counting Silver Linings, and by seven thirty in the morning I already had two!

I went home to sleep off my Valium buzz before my eleven thirty doctor's appointment (to which I asked my girlfriend to come). At this point I had finally learned *not* to go to a doctor's office without a friend! Well, my head had barely hit the pillow when my surgeon's office called to ask whether I would come an hour earlier so "we can have more time to talk." This was yet another bad sign. "Sure," I said, "we will be there."

We arrived promptly at the newly designated time and were escorted almost immediately to my surgeon's office. Isn't it a wonderful Silver Lining when physicians are on time? My Valium buzz was long gone. I was ready—well, as ready as I could possibly be—between my computer, for my notes, and a journal, for my girlfriend to take notes. I planned to record as much information as possible.

So there we were, ready. My surgeon calmly and gently said exactly what I expected her to say, "As I suspected, you do have breast cancer."

We spent more than an hour discussing breast cancer in general and my specific type, infiltrating ductal carcinoma. Infiltrating ductal carcinoma is the type of cancer that begins in the milk ducts but has grown into the surrounding normal breast tissue. This is the type of cancer that can spread to the lymph nodes (we wouldn't know if mine had spread until after surgery). Ductal carcinoma in situ (DCIS) is the type of cancer that stays inside

> ### LIFELINE
>
> *When you hear the words "You have breast cancer," do not make any rash decisions! Stop. Breathe. Think. A diagnosis is not an emergency (though it feels like it is!).*

> ### LIFELINE
>
> *With invasive ductal carcinoma, you are NOT alone. Of the more than two hundred thousand breast cancer diagnoses, about 80 percent are invasive ductal carcinomas.*

the milk ducts and doesn't spread into any normal surrounding breast tissue.

My surgeon went on to tell me that I was not a candidate for breast conservation therapy and that I should have a simple mastectomy with sentinel lymph node mapping and biopsy. All of a sudden, after the news of the diagnosis set in, I didn't really hear anything.

Here's the thing: even though I'm a nurse and have a fair amount of experience with cancer patients, when my surgeon was talking to me, it still sounded like Charlie Brown's teacher. All I heard was "*Whaa-whaa-whaa.*" The Silver Lining was that I had my laptop computer, and my girlfriend had a journal so we both took notes as she was talking.

My first question was, "What stage am I?" My surgeon said that we would not know my official "stage" until after surgery. Please allow me to back up a bit. A staging system provides a standardized method for determining whether the cancer has spread within the breast or to other parts of the body.

Determining a stage involves multiple steps, beginning with *clinical staging* (which is what I just had done with this surgeon). Clinical staging includes a biopsy, physical exam, and, sometimes, additional blood or imaging tests. The next step is surgery (either lumpectomy or mastectomy) to determine whether the cancer has spread. The results of the pathology tests done with the tissue collected during surgery would determine my stage. So, I wouldn't know the official diagnosis until after surgery.

I then asked her about the lesions in the left breast. "Because they are so hard to reach," she said, "we would need to do an MRI-guided breast biopsy to determine what those are." *Oy.*

She went on to tell me that because of my young age and that because my cancer was invasive, after surgery I would most likely need chemotherapy for four months and radiation for six weeks. I heard *that. Gulp.* All that kept running through my head was LiFT's mantra: We. Know. How. To. Do. This.

On a side note, as a hospice nurse and social worker, I have had to deliver a whole lot of bad news in my career, and I have to say that another

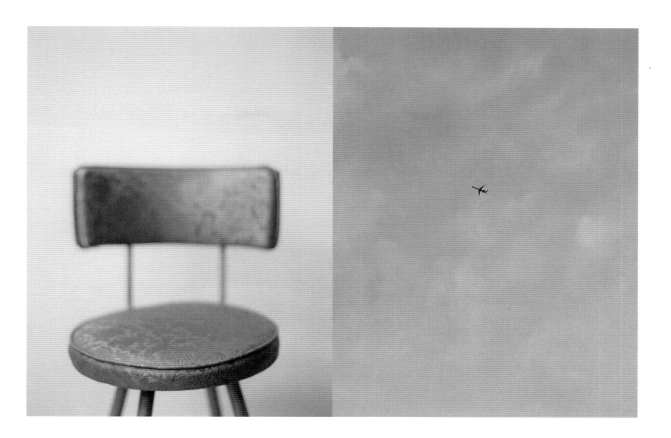

Silver Lining of this whole mess was that my surgeon did an incredible job of informing me that I had breast cancer. For the record, I know how strange that must be to read. It was even stranger to write.

This was Friday. My exhausted and worried husband landed in LA at about the time we finished meeting with the doctor. He had a ninety-minute drive home. So in the meantime, my girlfriend and I went out to lunch to process the news.

After lunch, I went home to wait for my husband. After flying thirty of the previous forty-eight hours (with a good eight hours spent in airport terminals), he finally rolled into the driveway. I'd never been happier to see anyone in my life. I imagine that there were a few tears when we embraced, but definitely no snot fest. We are both problem solvers and now we had a big, bad problem that needed a plan.

We were both pretty numb and exhausted and decided to take the day to rest. Quite frankly, I don't remember much of the rest of the day. The stress of this breast cancer diagnosis wiped out my memory bank.

LIFELINE

Studies suggest that even before treatment begins people may have mental fog & fatigue that result in problems with memory & concentration.

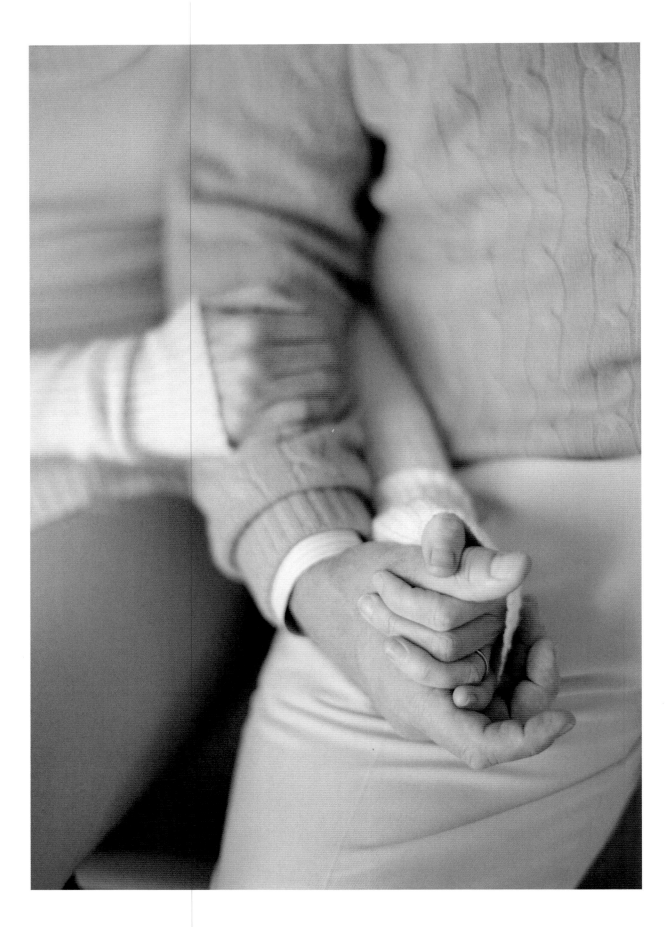

COMMUNICATING THE NEWS

When we came out of our fog—sort of—the first thing on our list of things to do was to tell family and friends the news. When it came to communicating the news about my diagnosis, I felt overwhelmed and decided that I just didn't have the capacity to call everyone who needed to know. Now the Silver Lining was that I had a wonderfully long list of people to tell.

Additionally, I also decided—as a wee bit of a control freak—that I wanted everyone to hear the news directly from me, in my own words. Hence, sending a group email was the best choice for me. What I didn't anticipate was the response: hundreds of emails asking "Is this a joke?" and "What stage are you?" and "What can I do?" and "How is this possible?" These emails, though lovingly intended, gave me a panic attack because I had no clue how I would muster the energy to respond to each and every one. So, I decided that rather than sending individual emails, communicating in a group format—via a blog—was going to be the best option. Hence *The Silver Pen* blog was born.

After my diagnosis, an innumerable number of people posed the *Why?* question to me. "How is it," they wondered, "that someone who is as healthy and fit and happy as you gets diagnosed with cancer?" Asking why is a common and natural response to nonsensical circumstances that are an inherent part of life. Despite the fact that my life was interrupted in the most abrupt and dastardly of ways, I didn't really question my diagnosis, at least not in that philosophical and deep way.

It's not to say that I haven't ever asked the big *Why?* question in life, because I certainly have. Many times. For example when a dear friend died recently (after having been diagnosed with stage IV cancer only nine months previously), I certainly asked *Why?* I also had many *Why?* questions when I was a pediatric hospice nurse caring for dying children. After all, the death of a child is the most unnatural circumstance in this world, for which there is absolutely no rational explanation.

However, after my diagnosis, I found myself in a surprisingly good place. I acknowledged that there were no readily apparent answers to the *Why?* question, so instead of wondering, "Why me?" I decided to proactively formulate a plan for coping with and managing the diagnosis and my attitude toward it.

I felt like I was exactly where I was supposed to be. No, I was not in denial and I don't think I was crazy. I did, however, feel like I was at an intangible height of emotional bring-it-on-ness. ♥

THE SILVER LINING

The Silver Lining is when inexplicable tragedy creates an **opportunity** to take righteous anger and sadness and turn them into a **force** for **finding the positives** in life. No, it's not easy. I would never suggest otherwise. What I do know for sure is that dumbfounding circumstances can be channeled into action that yields **positive** outcomes.

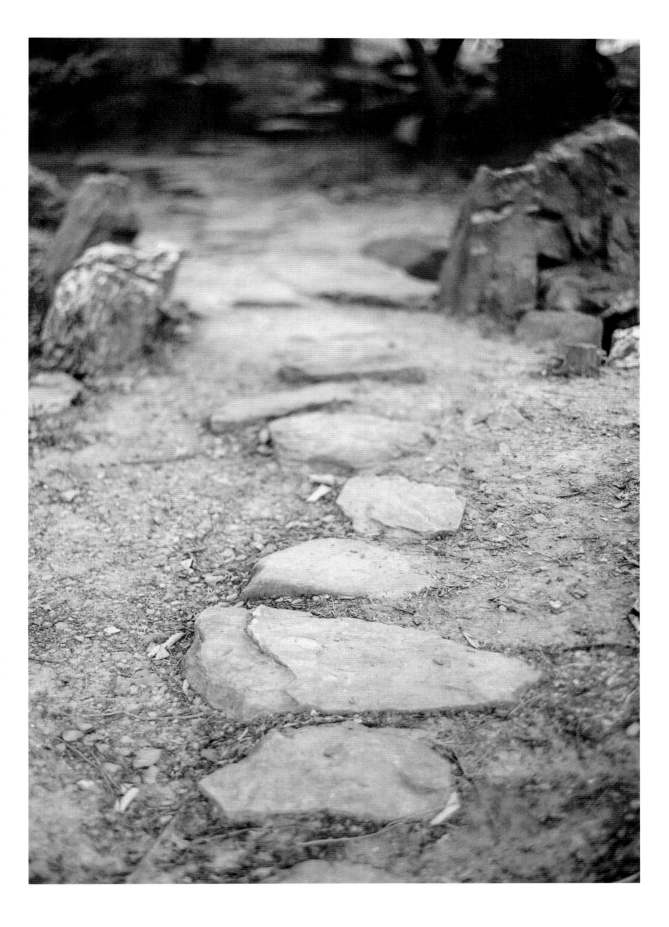

When Facing a Potential Diagnosis

1. Many doctors insist on waiting for full pathology reports before making an official diagnosis. This can result in a very long and anxiety-ridden waiting period. I can't tell you not to worry because that would be absurd. What I will recommend, however, is to engage your inner Zen-ny (think: *Om*) to calm your mind, body, and spirit. And breathe.

2. If you sense that something is wrong and a mammogram doesn't show anything, be your own advocate and insist on another test (e.g., ultrasound or MRI). Trust your instinct and intuition. No one knows your body better than you!

3. Always take a levelheaded, clear-thinking person with you to an appointment. She or he not only will be another set of ears but also will support you during this difficult experience.

4. Any time you go to a doctor's office for an important meeting, it is always very important to take as detailed notes as possible. Typically, people only hear a fraction of what is said in these types of anxiety-filled meetings. The benefit of taking notes, in addition to accumulating valuable information, is that it slows the conversation and allows you to ask clarifying questions.

5. After processing (to the best of your ability!) the information from your diagnosis appointment, begin a list of questions that you would like to have clarified and take that to your next appointment.

6. Humor is a very effective coping mechanism, even when laughter comes at seemingly awkward times.

7. Take a physician-prescribed pre-MRI sedative only *after* you confirm that the MRI machine is working!

8. Prior to any test or procedure, have the technician explain everything in detail, including the fact that MRIs are *loud*! Earplugs help diminish the noise.

9. It's normal to wonder, "Why did this happen to me?" However, after you ask the question, I encourage you to cease looking for answers, because there aren't any. Instead, I recommend that you start thinking proactively.

10. Learn everything that you can possibly learn about your type of breast cancer. However, resist the urge to blindly search the Internet for information. Instead, ask your physician for resources or turn to trusted resources such as breastcancer.org, the American Cancer Society, the National Cancer Institute, and Susan G. Komen for the Cure to understand your disease and begin to look at treatment options.

11. Do not make any rash decisions. Despite your feeling as if a bomb has hit you, the situation is not emergent (i.e., requiring medical intervention within twenty-four hours of diagnosis). Now is a time to be proactive rather than reactive; wait to make decisions until after you have had time to process the news.

12. Determine the best way for *you* to communicate with friends, family, and work colleagues about your diagnosis and upcoming treatment. Now is the time when you get to call the shots. *You* determine what is best for *you*.

13. Begin building your own comprehensive medical record. You legally own your medical records, so you cannot be refused access to them. At the time of every test, request a copy of the results and the progress notes written by nurses and physicians. Hospitals and clinics do have the right to charge you for these records, but it is well worth the investment. Take your medical record to each appointment.

14. Look for Silver Linings. Even on the darkest days, you will find them. All you have to do is look.

Medical Tests
(Not everyone has all tests)

BREAST PHYSICAL EXAM: Your doctor will assess both of your breasts, feeling for any lumps or other abnormalities, likely doing so in varying positions, such as with your arms above your head and at your side.

MAMMOGRAM: A mammogram is an X-ray of the breast used to screen for breast cancer. If an abnormality is seen, your doctor may recommend a diagnostic mammogram. This is a more detailed look at any suspicious area in your breasts that may be partially hidden due to naturally occurring lumps or dense breast tissue.

BREAST ULTRASOUND: The ultrasound uses high-frequency sound waves to create images of the breast and specifically suspicious spots in the breast. Ultrasounds cannot detect the presence of cancer; however, they can tell your doctor whether a suspicious area is solid (such as a benign lump or cancer), filled with fluid (such as a cyst), or a combination. A breast ultrasound may also be helpful in guiding a radiologic biopsy to get a sample of breast tissue if a solid mass is found. No radiation is used.

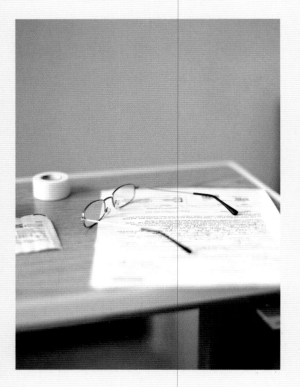

BREAST BIOPSY: The procedure to remove and evaluate a tissue sample to confirm the presence of cancer. A biopsy is done by placing a needle through the skin into the breast to remove a sample of tissue. There are different types of biopsies, including fine needle aspiration, core needle, vacuum-assisted, incisional, and excisional. It takes from several days to a week to get the (pathology) results. The waiting is *so hard*!

MAGNETIC RESONANCE IMAGING (MRI): A test that confirms a suspicious mass discovered in a screening mammogram, ultrasound, or clinical examination. An MRI uses magnets and radio waves to produce images of the interior of your breast. Before a breast MRI, you will receive an injection of dye into your veins. This test gives a sense of the extent of the cancer and shows whether there's any evidence of cancer in the other breast. In some cases, a diagnostic MRI may be appropriate in identifying possible cancers. MRIs do not use radiation.

CHEST X-RAY: A chest X-ray is a test used to determine whether the cancer has spread to your lungs and to assess the heart's and lung's capacity to handle treatment.

BONE SCAN: This imaging test uses radioactive material infused intravenously to determine the baseline health of your bones and whether the cancer has spread to the bones.

BLOOD TESTS: Blood tests are taken from the time of diagnosis throughout recovery. After diagnosis, your blood is assessed for circulating tumor cells to indicate whether the cancer has spread. Blood is taken throughout treatment as a way to analyze how well your body is handling the treatment and also to see whether the cancer is responding to the treatment. After treatment, your blood is analyzed for recurrence (i.e., whether the cancer has come back). I have frequent-flier miles at our local lab.

DIGITAL TOMOSYNTHESIS: A new type of screening test that takes 3-dimensional x-ray images of each breast from multiple angles. The Silver Linings are that it is more comfortable than a traditional mammogram, a lower dose of radiation is used, and the results are more comprehensive because it provides better visualization. Many clinicians anticipate that this procedure will replace mammography.

COMPUTED TOMOGRAPHY (CT) SCAN: A sophisticated X-ray that allows doctors to see detailed cross-sectional images of your internal organs. The test requires that dye be put into your arm intravenously. This dye makes your organs easier to see but can negatively affect your kidneys, which is why kidney function tests may be performed before giving you the contrast solution. In the world of breast cancer, one thing always seems to lead to another!

POSITRON EMISSION TOMOGRAPHY/POSITRON EMISSION MAMMOGRAPHY (PET/PEM): This test can detect areas of cancer by obtaining images of the body's cells as they work. You are injected with a substance made up of sugar and radioactive material. Cancer cells absorb more of the radioactive sugar than normal cells. Then you lie on a table and the scanner picks up certain areas of concern more clearly. I had a PET/PEM scan after I was done with treatment and thankfully, it showed no signs of breast cancer anywhere in my body, which was a *major* Silver Lining!

BRCA1 AND BRCA2 TESTS: BRCA1 and BRCA2 are genetic tests that identify a potential link to hereditary breast and ovarian cancer. A woman's risk of developing breast and/or ovarian cancer is increased if she inherits a BRCA1 or BRCA2 mutation. Note: this does not—in any way, shape, or form—guarantee a breast cancer diagnosis. Rather, it increases a person's risk. I am BRCA1 and BRCA2 negative.

For more information, please go to breastcancer.org.

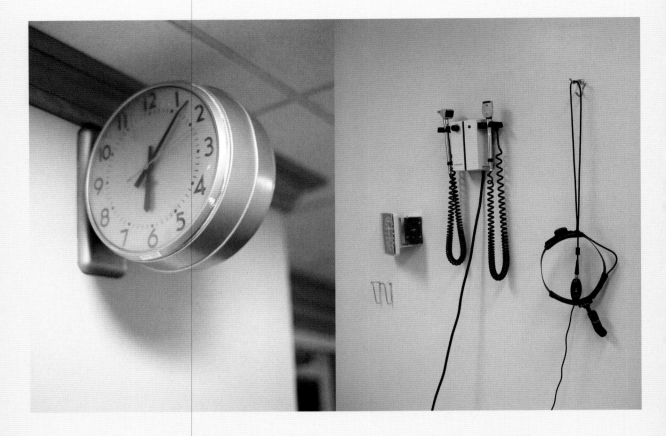

Coping Mechanisms for Needle Phobia

- Tell the phlebotomist (the person who draws your blood) or your nurse that you have needle phobia.

- Look away or close your eyes. If you're frightened, why torture yourself by watching?

- Take deep breaths, especially when the needle punctures your skin.

- Allow a maximum of two sticks per person. Hold your ground. Tell the person, "I have a two-stick-maximum policy. I'd like another phlebotomist, please."

- Request a butterfly needle. It is the smallest needle available and just as effective.

- For especially difficult veins, you can request a topical numbing agent (though not all labs have them).

- Busy your mind by counting backward from some unreasonable number that will actually make you think as you count down (e.g., 1,359,112).

- Don't chat with the phlebotomist. It is important for the person taking aim at your veins to be fully focused on the task at hand.

Questions to Ask Your Doctor About Testing

1. What is the purpose of the test or procedure?
2. What is involved with this particular medical test or procedure?
3. Is the test or procedure urgent (i.e., does it need to be done within twenty-four hours)?
4. Are there any other options for the test or procedure?
5. What is the cost? Will my insurance cover it?
6. Does the test or procedure require hospitalization or can it be done outpatient?
7. What are the potential side effects or risks of the test?
8. Will the test confirm a diagnosis?
9. When can I expect my test results?
10. Will I receive my test results face-to-face or by phone?
11. What do the test results actually mean in terms of diagnosis, treatment, and prognosis?
12. What is my risk of breast cancer?

Questions to Ask Your Doctor at the Time of Diagnosis

1. What type of breast cancer do I have? What is my exact diagnosis?
2. Can the stage of my breast cancer be determined?
3. Would you explain my pathology report to me?
4. May I have a copy of my pathology report and your doctor notes for my records?
5. Do I have a genetic mutation (BRCA1 or BRCA2)?
6. Do I need any more tests?
7. Has the cancer metastasized (spread to any other site)? If so, where?
8. What treatment options are available for me?
9. What is the timing of the treatments?
10. How quickly do I need to make a decision about cancer treatment?
11. What are the benefits and potential side effects of each treatment you recommend?
12. Will treatments affect my fertility? If so, what can I do before beginning treatment?
13. Is there one treatment you recommend over the others?
14. How will each treatment affect my daily life?
15. Can I work during treatment?
16. What will cancer treatment cost?
17. Do you have any oncology or surgical doctor referrals?
18. Will my insurance cover second opinions and treatment?
19. Where can I learn more about my diagnosis (e.g., websites and books)?
20. What support services do you recommend?
21. What is my hormone receptor status?

Staging*

Breast cancer stage is determined by:

- the site of the tumor
- the size of the tumor
- whether the cancer is invasive or noninvasive
- whether cancer cells have spread to lymph nodes under your arm
- whether cancer cells have spread to other parts of your body

Breast cancer staging systems continue to evolve as new scientific research on cancer emerges. Some staging systems are useful for several types of cancer; others are relevant only for particular types of cancer. The TNM (tumor, node, and metastasis) staging system, accepted by the American Joint Committee on Cancer (AJCC) and the Union for International Cancer Control (UICC), is the most widely used breast cancer staging system. The National Cancer Institute's database also uses the TNM system.

The TNM system is based upon:

- *T* for tumor size
- *N* for lymph node involvement
- *M* for metastases or spread of cancer from one part of the body to another
- The letter *X* indicates that the tumor cannot be evaluated.

The letters *is* refer to carcinoma "in situ," which describes a cancer that is only present in the cells where it started and has not spread to surrounding tissue.

In addition to the letter, a number corresponds to either the size of the tumor or the extent to which the cancer has spread. The letter *T* is followed by a number from 0 to 4, the letter *N* is followed by a number from 0 to 3, and the letter *M* is followed by a 0 or 1 when using the TNM staging system.

The TNM staging system is as follows:

- TX: Primary tumor cannot be evaluated.
- T0: No evidence of primary tumor.
- Tis: Abnormal cells are present but have not spread.
- T1: Tumor is 2 centimeters (¾ inch) or less.
- T2: Tumor is more than 2 centimeters but not more than 5 centimeters (2 inches).
- T3: Tumor is more than 5 centimeters.
- T4: Tumor is any size and has spread into neighboring tissue.

For more information, go to the National Cancer Institute website: cancer.gov.

- NX: Lymph nodes cannot be evaluated.
- N0: Cancer has not spread to lymph nodes.
- N1: Cancer has spread to one to three axillary (underarm) lymph nodes, and/or small amounts of cancer are found in internal mammary lymph nodes (near the breastbone).
- N2: Cancer has spread to four to nine axillary or internal mammary lymph nodes.
- N3: Cancer has spread to either the axillary or internal lymph nodes with at least one area greater than 2 millimeters.
- MX: Distant metastasis cannot be found or measured.
- M0: No distant metastasis.
- M1: Distant metastasis is present (spread to distant organs such as bone, brain, liver, or lungs).

Once determined, the data from the T, N, and M categories can be combined with another system of breast cancer staging called *stage grouping*. Sometimes used alone, breast cancer stage grouping is recorded with a number ranging from 0 to Roman numeral IV, with many subcategories. Lower numbers indicate earlier stages of cancer, while higher numbers reflect late-stage cancers:

STAGE 0 (INCLUDES TIS, N0, M0): Describes noninvasive breast cancer where there is no evidence of cancer cells or noncancerous abnormal cells spreading beyond the breast.

STAGE I: An early stage of invasive breast cancer where cancer cells are invading normal surrounding breast tissue.

- stage IA (includes T1, N0, M0): The tumor measures up to 2 centimeters and no lymph nodes are involved.

- stage IB (includes T0, T1, some N1s, M0): Cancer cells that are larger than 0.2 millimeters but not larger than 2 millimeters exist in the lymph nodes, with either no tumor in the breast or the tumor is 2 centimeters or smaller.

STAGE II: Indicates invasive breast cancer cells.

- stage IIA (includes T0, T1, T2, some N1s, M0): The tumor is larger than 2 centimeters but not larger than 5 centimeters and has not spread to the lymph nodes, *or* the tumor is 2 centimeters or smaller and also found in the lymph nodes *or* no tumor is found in the breast but cancer cells are found in the lymph nodes under the arm.

- stage IIB (includes T2, T3, N0, N1, M0): The tumor is larger than 2 centimeters but not larger than 5 centimeters and cancer cells larger than 0.2 millimeters but not larger than 2 millimeters are found in the lymph nodes, *or* the tumor is larger than 2 centimeters but not larger than 5 centimeters and cancer cells have spread to one, two, or three lymph nodes under the arm or near the breastbone *or* the tumor is larger than

5 centimeters and has not spread to lymph nodes. This is where I landed because I had lymph node involvement.

STAGE III: Indicates an invasive stage of cancer that has not spread to distant body organs.

- stage IIIA (includes T0, T2, T3, N1, N2, M0): The tumor is larger than 5 centimeters and the cancer has spread to one, two, or three lymph nodes under the arm or near the breastbone *or* the tumor is larger than 5 centimeters and small clusters of cancer cells larger than 0.2 millimeters but not larger than 2 millimeters are found in the lymph nodes *or* no tumor is found in the breast or it may be any size and cancer is found in four to nine lymph nodes under the arm or near the breastbone.

- stage IIIB (includes T4, N0, N2, M0): The tumor may be any size and cancer cells have spread to the chest wall and/or skin of the breast and possibly the lymph nodes within the breast, under the arm, or near the breastbone.

- stage IIIC (includes any T, N3, M0): No tumor is found or the tumor may be any size and the cancer cells may have spread to the chest wall and/or skin of the breast *and/or* spread to ten or more lymph nodes under the arm *and/or* lymph nodes above or below the collarbone and near the neck.

STAGE IV (INCLUDES ANY T, ANY N, M1): Describes invasive breast cancer that has spread outside the breast and lymph nodes to distant parts of the body such as the bones, lungs, liver, or brain. The words "advanced" and "metastatic" are used to describe stage IV breast cancer, either at the time of the initial diagnosis or when a previous cancer has spread.

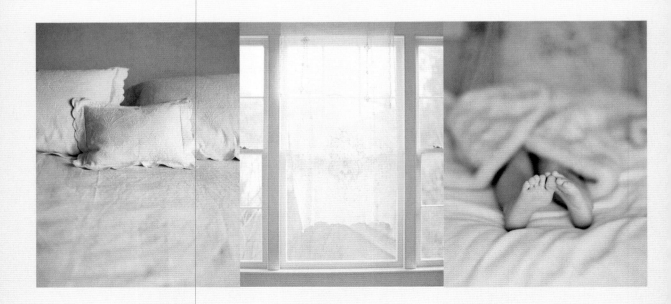

Different Types of Breast Cancer*

DUCTAL CARCINOMA IN SITU (DCIS): "Carcinoma" refers to any cancer that initially develops in the skin or other tissues, including breast tissue. "In situ," meaning "in the original place," describes a cancer that is only present in the cells where it started and has not spread to surrounding tissue. DCIS is considered the most common type of noninvasive breast cancer (about one out of five cases). With DCIS, abnormal cells are found in the lining of the breast milk ducts. Although DCIS is not life threatening, the diagnosis increases the risk of cancer reoccurrence; however, the chances are less than 30 percent without radiation and 15 percent with radiation. About a 50 percent chance exists of the cancer being invasive should there be a reoccurrence.

INVASIVE DUCTAL CARCINOMA (IDC): With IDC, cancerous cells are found in the lining of the breast milk ducts and also found invading the surrounding tissue. Undetected, invasive ductal carcinoma can spread to the lymph nodes and/or possibly other organs in the body. Seventy to eighty percent of all breast cancer diagnoses are IDC, making it the most common type. IDC is also the most common type of breast cancer to affect men. Of the women diagnosed with IDC, about two-thirds are over the age of fifty-five.

TUBULAR CARCINOMA OF THE BREAST (IDC TYPE): As a subtype of invasive ductal carcinoma, tubular carcinoma of the breast is also found inside of the breast milk ducts and invading the surrounding tissue. Tubular carcinomas are generally small (1 centimeter or less), distinctive tube-shaped structures (referred to as "tubules") that make up a cluster of cells that feel "spongy" under the breast tissue rather than like a lump. Making up about 2 percent of all breast cancer diagnoses, tubular carcinoma is found mostly in women in their early fifties and is rare in men. Although invasive, this type of breast cancer is typically less aggressive and responds well to hormone therapy.

MEDULLARY CARCINOMA OF THE BREAST (IDC TYPE): Considered a rare subtype of invasive ductal carcinoma, medullary carcinoma of the breast gets its name from its soft, fleshy consistency, which resembles a part in the brain called the medulla. Like tubular carcinoma, medullary carcinoma feels "spongy" under the breast tissue rather than like a lump. Making up about 3 to 5 percent of all breast cancer cases, medullary carcinoma cells look aggressive; however, they grow slowly and seldom spread outside the breast into the lymph nodes. Found more frequently in women in Japan than in the United States, medullary carcinoma typically responds well to treatment.

MUCINOUS CARCINOMA OF THE BREAST (IDC TYPE): Considered a rare subtype of invasive ductal carcinoma, mucinous carcinoma of the breast gets its name from being made up of cancerous cells that "float" in a slimy, slippery substance called mucin (a key ingredient in

Adapted from breastcancer.org, used with permission.

mucus). About 2 to 3 percent of invasive breast cancers are considered 100 percent mucinous carcinoma of the breast. About 5 percent of invasive breast cancer diagnoses contain a mucinous component. Women diagnosed with mucinous carcinoma tend to be in their sixties or seventies, and men are rarely diagnosed with this type of breast cancer. Although invasive, mucinous carcinoma is less aggressive and has a favorable prognosis in most cases.

PAPILLARY CARCINOMA OF THE BREAST (IDC TYPE): Considered a rare subtype of invasive ductal carcinoma, papillary carcinoma of the breast gets its name from being made up of cancerous cells that are arranged in fingerlike projections, or papules. This type of breast cancer accounts for less than 1 to 2 percent of all breast cancers; men are occasionally diagnosed with this type, and most women diagnosed have already gone through menopause. Papillary carcinoma of the breast generally has a favorable prognosis.

CRIBRIFORM CARCINOMA OF THE BREAST (IDC TYPE): A type of invasive ductal carcinoma in which cancerous cells invade the stroma, or connective tissues of the breast. Nestlike formations between the ducts and lobules are created once invaded by the abnormal cells. The tumor is said to resemble Swiss cheese because of the distinctive punched-out holes in between the cancerous cells.

INVASIVE LOBULAR CARCINOMA (ILC): Also referred to as infiltrating lobular carcinoma. ILC diagnoses make up 10 percent of all invasive breast cancers, making it the second most common type of breast cancer. Invasive lobular carcinoma is generally diagnosed in women in their sixties. Research suggests that hormone replacement therapy may increase the risk of this type of breast cancer.

INFLAMMATORY BREAST CANCER (IBC): Considered a rare and aggressive type of breast cancer, IBC accounts for 1 to 5 percent of all breast cancer cases. Rather than by a lump, IBC is usually detected by reddening and swelling of the breast that may feel warm to the touch. IBC often goes undetected on a mammogram due to the absence of a lump. The breast affected by IBC may become more firm, itchy, tender, or large. IBC is known to grow and spread extremely rapidly; seeking prompt treatment is imperative. Inflammatory breast cancer tends to be more common in African American women. This aggressive type of breast cancer has a greater chance of spreading quickly and a bleaker prognosis than typical invasive or ductal or lobular cancer.

LOBULAR CARCINOMA IN SITU (LCIS): With LCIS, abnormal cells develop in the lobules, or milk-producing glands, located at the ends of the breast ducts. Usually more than one lobule is affected. Lobular carcinoma in situ involves one or more areas of abnormal cell growth, which indicates a higher-than-average risk for developing breast cancer in the future; therefore, it is not a "true" breast cancer. Some professionals prefer the term "lobular neoplasia" instead of "lobular carcinoma" for this reason. LCIS is generally diagnosed in women before menopause and is extremely uncommon in men.

PAGET'S DISEASE OF THE NIPPLE: Considered a rare form of breast cancer, Paget's disease (also known as mammary Paget's disease) accounts for only 1 percent of all breast cancer cases. Cancer cells gather in and around the nipple and areola, often making the area crusty, irritated, itchy, red, and scaly, with bleeding and oozing not uncommon. Paget's disease is frequently an indication that either DCIS or invasive cancer exists elsewhere in the breast. Although more common in women, Paget's disease can also affect men.

PHYLLODES TUMORS OF THE BREAST: This type of tumor develops in the stoma (connective tissue) and accounts for only 1 percent of all breast tumors. "Phyllodes" is a Greek term meaning "leaflike," and refers to the leaflike pattern created by the cell growth. Although the cells are known to grow quickly, they rarely spread outside the breast. Phyllodes tumors can be benign, malignant, or borderline. They usually develop in women in their forties and are extremely rare in men.

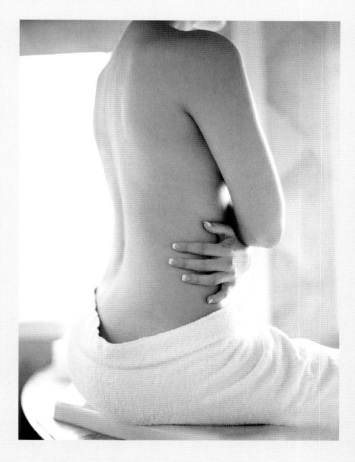

TRIPLE-NEGATIVE BREAST CANCER: With this type of cancer, the three most common types of receptors known to fuel breast cancer growth are lacking: estrogen, progesterone, and the HER2/neu gene. This makes common treatments like hormone therapy and certain drugs that target these receptors ineffective. Triple-negative breast cancer grows and spreads quickly; however, especially in its early stages, it responds well to chemotherapy. Triple-negative breast cancer tends to occur more frequently in younger and African American women.

METASTATIC BREAST CANCER: This type of cancer has spread to other parts of the body and may include the bones, brain, liver, and/or lungs. The cancer may spread in various ways, including (1) healthy cells are invaded by cancer cells, (2) the circulatory or lymph cells are penetrated by cancer cells, (3) the bloodstream or lymph system transports the cancer cells, (4) cancer cells stop moving and get lodged in the capillaries, and (5) new tumors develop in new locations.

CHAPTER II

Children Always Know

Communicating with Children About a Cancer Diagnosis

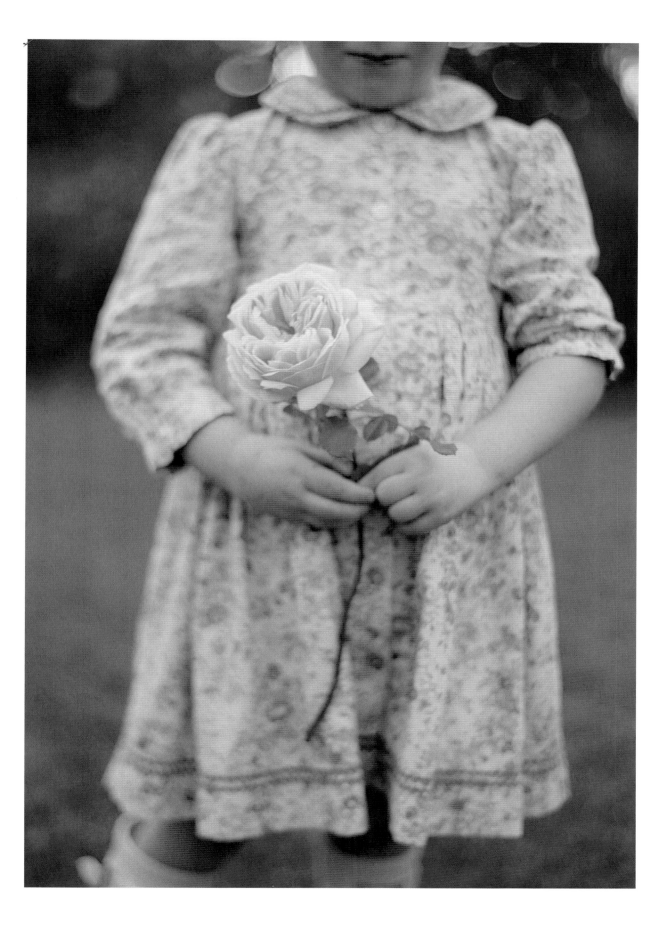

We have four children in our family, three young adult men and a daughter, who, at the time of my diagnosis, was four and three-quarters. As much as I wish this experience only happened to me and that I could have shielded my husband and children from the pain, the reality is that cancer does not happen in isolation. Cancer happens within the ecosystem of family, friends, and community.

In my professional experience as a pediatric hospice nurse and social worker, I have seen firsthand that children always know something serious is going on even when no one says anything to them. Children are incredibly intuitive and observant; we adults simply do not give them enough credit. From the time of a diagnosis, children are keenly aware that something major has happened in their family and try immediately (either on their own or, hopefully, with adult assistance) to make sense of and cope with the situation.

Children deserve to know what is happening. Silence is *not* golden. Really, it isn't. What children need most in this life is to know what is true and the wisdom and guidance to help make sense of things. When facing a cancer diagnosis, talking about illness candidly and openly, in developmentally appropriate ways, demonstrates that parents are trustworthy and that truthfulness is a family priority. When children are young, we can deny or think that they won't understand, but that doesn't keep them safe, and it doesn't make their childhood happy.

Now, this acknowledgment certainly doesn't discount how challenging it is to tell your child(ren) about a life-rocking situation. Telling children of any age about a cancer diagnosis is incredibly challenging and certainly very emotional. The Silver Lining is that there are resources to help include and guide your children through the breast cancer experience.

AVOIDANCE

So why do some adults avoid talking with children? Many loving, intelligent, and responsible parents find themselves trying to hide the truth from children because they think: "Children don't understand what is happening." That is pure and utter malarkey. Children as young as a year know when things are haywire in a household, whether it is due to divorce or illness. They *know*.

Another common reason why adults avoid telling children is that they think they shouldn't be exposed to something so awful. Well, that's one hundred percent true. Exposing children to cancer is brutal and heartbreaking. For me, telling our children was the hardest part of the whole breast cancer experience. However, life inevitably has its way of throwing us some hefty challenges. The best way to handle these challenges, no matter how dire, is head-on. Denial, though it may feel like the correct course at first, only exacerbates the pain of the circumstances.

For those people who have a challenging time talking with children about difficult things, like cancer, please keep in mind that no matter how hard adults try to hide information, whatever is being discussed in the house (even behind closed doors) *will* be overheard and felt by the children. When they don't hear the whole story and don't

understand what they do hear, they are likely to be confused. This confusion can easily turn into fear.

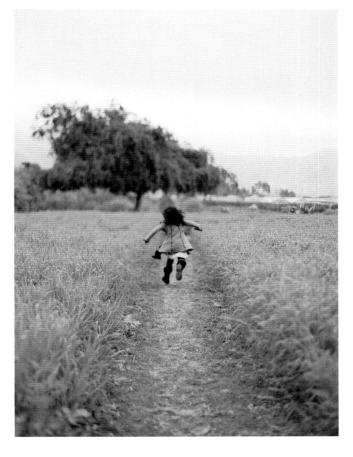

When children are given the message that breast cancer (or any other catastrophic event) shouldn't be discussed, they don't discuss it. Therefore, when children are left alone with upsetting, inaccurate information, they consequently suffer alone in silence. This solitude forces them to draw their own conclusions and/or find maladaptive ways of dealing with a loved one's cancer diagnosis. How awful is that?

A child's imagination has the capacity to create things far worse than the reality. No matter what children are told, they can come up with something that is much more awful. It sounds hard to believe, but it's true. I've seen it happen time and again and it's sad, so sad.

Furthermore, if children catch you in a lie of omission or deception (even when lovingly intended), then from that point forward, they will always wonder, "Are Mommy and Daddy not telling me something?" Avoidance may feel better in the short term, but it has the potential to do long-term damage. Getting the theme here?

In a nutshell, including children in the disease diagnosis and treatments (using developmentally appropriate language), though emotionally burdensome and painful, will ultimately be the greatest gift that parents can give. The words, actions, trust, and love in the lives of children will determine their ability to cope with the illness.

DELIVERING THE NEWS

After we gathered as much information about my situation as we possibly could, including my diagnosis and plan for surgery (at the time we were not one hundred percent certain that I would need to have chemotherapy and radiation), it was time to tell the kids. When it came to communicating with our children, feelings of anxiety and sadness spewed in unimaginable ways.

When I was working as a pediatric hospice nurse and I met a family for the first time, I would always say to the parents, "Now, I know that this is a ridiculously dumb question, but what is your biggest concern?" Two times out of ten, the parents would say, "Yes, that is the dumbest question I've ever heard. My child is dying." Eight times out of ten, however, they would say, "We don't know how to talk with our other children."

I now felt similar feelings of anxiety and had to give myself a *Moonstruck* "snap out of it" moment by reminding myself that after all of my clinical experience, there was no one more prepared to tell our children. However, I was still a nervous wreck. I was prepared to contend with my illness. I was not prepared for our children to contend with my illness.

Talk about irony. Suddenly, I was forced to follow the advice that in my clinical work I had dispensed so many times to so many patients over the years. Truth be told, for a split second, I wondered whether all of the advice I had given really works. There was only one way to find out.

The place to begin is with preparation. Prior to our conversation(s), my husband and I assessed which of our children to tell what and when. Because children absorb complex information at different levels, it is important to begin a discussion from where they are in their developmental process.

Because of their ages (twenty-seven, twenty-four, nineteen), we spoke openly and candidly with the boys. We knew that they had the capacity to understand clinical details and could cope with the uncertainties of my diagnosis and course of treatment. Because they lived in three different cities, we told each of the boys by phone, in the evening, after work and school. I would have preferred to tell them in person, but the phone was our best option at the time because it was very important for them to hear the news directly from us, rather than from another source.

Prior to our conversations with them, we wrote down bullet points of information

LIFELINE

Steps to prepare for the conversation with your child(ren):
1. Prepare talking points.
2. Begin at the child's developmental level.
3. Make time & space for reaction.

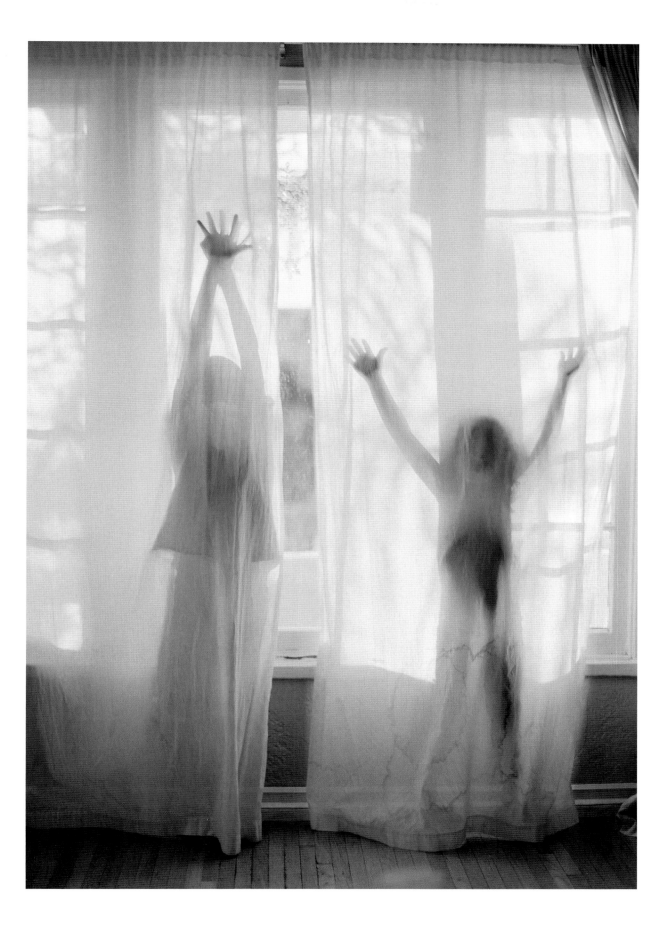

LIFELINE

*Prioritize open & honest
family communication.
It is imperative that your
child(ren) hear about
the diagnosis from you.*

to discuss to ensure that we could have as structured and complete a conversation as possible. Additionally, not knowing how each would react, we made sure that we cleared our schedule to allow each the time and space to respond as he needed. It's amazing, by the way, how a breast cancer diagnosis blows a calendar to pieces!

Each of them was stunned. They lovingly offered to drop everything and hop in a car or plane to be with us. We told them that this was going to be a very long process and that we would indeed need them, but that it would be better to wait until we knew our plans.

The approach we took with our young daughter, Lalee, was very different. At the time of my diagnosis, our daughter was an inquisitive, precocious, and sensitive preschooler. Typical features of this preschool stage of child development include:

- Egocentricity. In other words, "It's all about *me*." In the life of a preschooler, the majority of cause-and-effect events are seen only in relationship to them. (Don't you miss the good old days?)

- Associative logic. This means that any two unrelated things can be connected as if one causes or explains the other; for example, my sister wants a pony because she is a girl. Though this line of thinking doesn't make sense to us grown-ups, it is perfectly logical to a preschooler.

- Magical thinking. This is a typical aspect of preschool development in which children believe that their thoughts and actions directly influence or cause events around them. An example of magical thinking is, "It rained because I was thirsty."

- Play. It is the way children explore reality. It is how they acquire information and grow: physically, socially, intellectually, and emotionally. Tremendous insight can be gained by observing children while they are playing.

In my professional life as a pediatric nurse and social worker, I followed Kathleen McCue's recommendation in her book, *How to Help Children Through a Parent's Serious Illness,* to tell the children with whom I worked three things:

1. Mom or Dad is sick.
2. The name of the disease.
3. What may happen and what they can expect to see.

I applied this advice to the conversation we had with our daughter as well. To tell her, first I prepared by writing down these three things. Then, with my husband by my side, I sat on our bed and asked her to sit on my lap, facing me. I told her that we needed to have a serious talk. I asked her what "serious" meant (because I didn't want to make *any* assumptions that she knew or didn't know what words mean!) and she said "important." "Good," I thought, "she is totally focused."

Here is what I said and her responses:

1. *Me:* "I am sick."
   Lalee: She lowered her head and said, "I know. In your boobies." Note that I had *not* told her anything yet, but she still knew. I told her that she was right and that "boobies" are really called breasts (because we use anatomically correct language in our family).

2. *Me:* "My disease is called breast cancer."
   Lalee: "What is breast cancer and why did they get there?" Taking into account her developmental stage, I explained to her in appropriate terms (described later in the chapter) what cancer is. As to the question of "Why did they get there?" I told her the truth and said that we didn't know why and that some things in life, good and bad, just happen without any explanation.

3. *Me:* "I am going to be taken care of by nurses and doctors in a hospital for four nights."
   Lalee: "So what are the nurses and doctors going to do in the hospital?" I told her that they were going to put me into a very deep sleep and that they would cut the breast cancer cells out. "Is it going to hurt?" she asked worriedly. I said that I wouldn't feel anything because I would be in a deep sleep. She then asked, "Will Daddy wake you up with a magical kiss like Prince Charming woke up Sleeping Beauty?" For some reason, it was *that* question that really struck the emotional chord. With a shaky voice, I told her that the medicine would wear off and that I would wake up, and when I did, Daddy would be there to give me a magical kiss. And he did!

> **LIFELINE**
>
> *Don't make assumptions about what children know or don't know. Always ask them to both repeat what you say & explain it in their own words. Be patient until you are sure that they understand.*

QUESTIONS

LIFELINE

It is helpful to ask your children what they think caused the cancer. This way you can dispel the notion that they may have caused it. Additionally, reassure children that no one caused the cancer & that they will be cared for.

Also considering my clinical experience and Kathleen McCue's writing, I knew that at some point or another, there would be at least three questions Lalee would inevitably wonder, either out loud or in her mind: Did I cause the cancer? Is it contagious? Who will take care of me? I know it sounds unbelievable, but children really do think that they could have a role in causing cancer, that it is contagious, and that they might be left alone.

Children will inevitably bring up these questions whether they articulate them verbally or not. They will also likely want to know what cancer is and whether or not you are going to die from the disease. These are incredibly intense conversations, but if the dialogue doesn't happen, then a child is left alone with her own imagination. Don't assume that because children don't talk about something that isn't on their minds.

When we told Lalee about my diagnosis, we wanted to provide enough information to dispel her immediate fears, but also not overwhelm her with too much information. We reassured her that we would keep her informed and prepare her for what was coming next.

OPEN COMMUNICATION

After we told Lalee about the breast cancer diagnosis, we had an open line of communication throughout my entire treatment period and recovery. Because we did

LIFELINE

Keep in mind that being honest does not necessarily mean telling everything, especially when a child isn't ready to understand. It does, however, mean always telling the truth!

not want her to worry alone, we encouraged Lalee to talk with us about what she was thinking and feeling and to share with us what she may have heard about my illness, or about cancer in general, from other adults and children. The Silver Lining is that open and honest communication creates the opportunity to dispel unfounded worries.

We also encouraged Lalee to ask questions, as many as she wanted, whenever she wanted. Her list of questions went on and on and on and on, which was wonderful because it reflected her engagement and willingness to talk openly about it. Some of the questions that she asked over the days that followed included:

1. How will they cut your breast cancer out?
2. What kind of knife will they use?
3. Are you sure you will be asleep enough so you don't feel it?
4. Can you wear a princess dress during surgery?
5. What are your doctors' names?
6. What types of things are in a hospital?
7. What will be in your hospital room?
8. Will Daddy and Auntie LiFT (my BFF who stayed with me in the hospital) hold your hands to make you feel better?
9. How long will your breasts hurt?
10. Are you going to die?

Inevitably, the subject of death will come up. People do die from breast cancer. I happen to believe that I'm not going to be one of those people. The preschool age is the period in which children develop an age-appropriate fascination, bordering on obsession, with death. When this topic arises, as difficult as it may be, parents need to be completely open to answer questions honestly, without evasion or embarrassment. When our daughter asked me, my response was, "I don't think so and my doctors don't think so."

> **LIFELINE**
>
> *Children absorb information best when delivered in small doses. Delivering news slowly & thoughtfully will help in the understanding & digestion of the information.*

Some children may ask questions right away, like our daughter did, or they may need time to absorb the bomb that has just exploded in their lives. A general rule of thumb is to let children initiate conversations; however, a little prodding doesn't hurt. For example, you could ask: "Have you been thinking at all about Mommy's breast cancer?" If the answer is yes, follow up with, "What have you been wondering?"

Another question to elicit conversation is "What are you feeling about Mommy's breast cancer?" If children are willing to share emotions, allow them to flow. Do not stop the sometimes uncomfortable emotions of a child's sadness (that includes crying) or anger. These are healthy responses. Expression is so much better than their holding emotions inside only for them to be manifested later through other maladaptive behaviors. As difficult as it may be to witness such emotions in a child, it is important that we do so.

Another option would be to ask, "Do you have any questions that you would like to ask about Mommy's breast cancer?" If they say no to any of the questions, remind them: "You can ask me [or us] anything, anytime."

It is important not to force dialogue. Eventually, the thoughts and emotions *will*

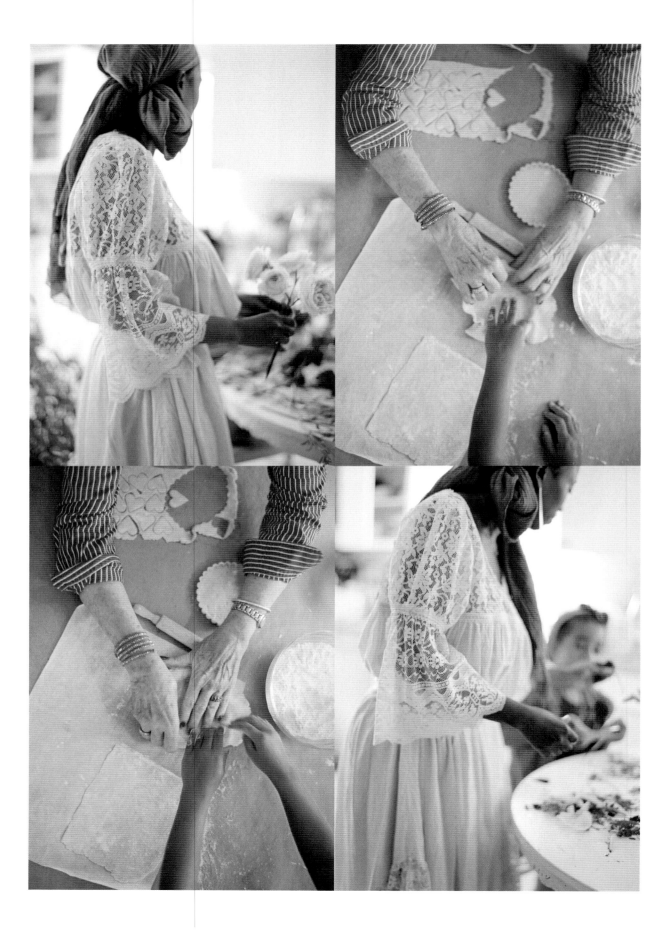

come. Allowing children to talk and share emotions on their own terms gives them a sense of control. When a child is encouraged to have an element of control in a seemingly uncontrollable situation, self-esteem and confidence develop. This lesson applies to life in general, not just during cancer treatment.

ROUTINE

In addition to our emphasis on open communication, we maintained a consistent schedule (e.g., bedtime routines) with normal discipline and limit setting just as we had before the diagnosis. Often, adults make errors of kindness. For example, they may allow children to stay up late to watch a movie or eat whatever they want because Mommy is sick. No! No! No! The best thing that we could do for our daughter was to keep her routines and life as normal and predictable as possible.

I have some pretty strident, evidence-based beliefs about sleep and diet: they are absolutely, positively the most important fundamentals of childhood. Without a good night of sleep, everything else goes haywire. As if after a breast cancer diagnosis things aren't already out of whack enough. No matter what: keep bedtime and eating routines normal-normal-normal. Routine is safe and comforting to a child. Of course, there are always special circumstances, but keep them just that—special.

SILVER LININGS

In addition to maintaining a consistent schedule, we taught Lalee about Silver Linings. I introduced the concept to her by describing a Silver Lining as seeing the good in something bad. Then, we sat down together and came up with a list of Silver Linings in our life as well as Silver Lining activities that we could do when I was sick. Creating this list was a Silver Lining in and of itself!

Lalee loves watching movies, so our first Silver Lining was developing a "Silver Lining Movie List." The list included all of her favorite movies that we intended to watch when I wasn't feeling well. The best part about this was that we could be together, doing something that she loved, without taxing my energy reserves.

Lalee is incredibly affectionate and happens to be a great hugger. Since I was not able to hug after my double mastectomy and reconstruction due to pain (which was incredibly heartbreaking, by the way), we came up with creative ways of showing love. "Leg Hugs" were one of my favorite gestures. Oh my goodness. Have you ever had one? If not, you must ask your child for a Leg Hug. They feel absolutely awesome!

Because Lalee loves to read, we also created a Silver Lining Book List. Incidentally, bibliotherapy is a wonderful expressive therapy that utilizes books and storytelling to help children cope with unsettling events in their lives. The written word, in the form of stories and poems, promotes emotional healing, calms fears, and enhances cognitive understanding.

Another Silver Lining activity was taking photographs together. After I was diagnosed, I bought a new camera (retail therapy?). I had always wanted to learn to take (good!) photographs, and during my postsurgical and chemotherapy-induced downtime, I had the opportunity. So every day, we walked, talked, and took Mommy-Daughter photographs together.

My favorite Silver Lining was the one called "Brother Adventures." When our boys asked what they could do to help, I asked them to comfort and support Lalee, by spending as much time with her (either in person or via technology) as possible.

One of the boys said, "Great. We'll have 'Brother Adventures' and help take care of her." I tear up just thinking about how much this meant to me, knowing that whenever Lalee needed extra love and strength, it would be there from her brothers.

Telling your child that you have breast cancer (or anything of that magnitude) is definitely an emotional experience. As if having breast cancer isn't hard enough. *Phew.* We cannot and need not shield children from our feelings completely. If you get emotional while talking with children, that's normal and okay. This is heavy-duty stuff we are talking about.

> ## LIFELINE
>
> *You are not alone. There is a great deal of professional support to help you talk with your children. You can ask your doctor, nurse, or social worker for assistance to help you in this process.*

The thing to do is to simply acknowledge to the children that parents sometimes feel scared, sad, angry, or worried, but that it won't last forever. Let your children know that it is okay for them to sometimes feel those things too. In fact, sharing a few tears together can reassure children that feelings do not need to be completely overwhelming, and that parents will be there to support them and to try to understand how they feel. Consider this a great opportunity to model coping behavior to children and to teach them to develop coping mechanisms in their own lives.

Trust the children in your life. Don't hide what you know to be true. When there is trust, you can survive anything and everything. The willingness to be truthful changes us—for the better. Keeping children safe is not to deny what is happening but to say "We. Can. Do. This." No matter what the "this" is. This sounds so much more difficult than it actually is. ♥

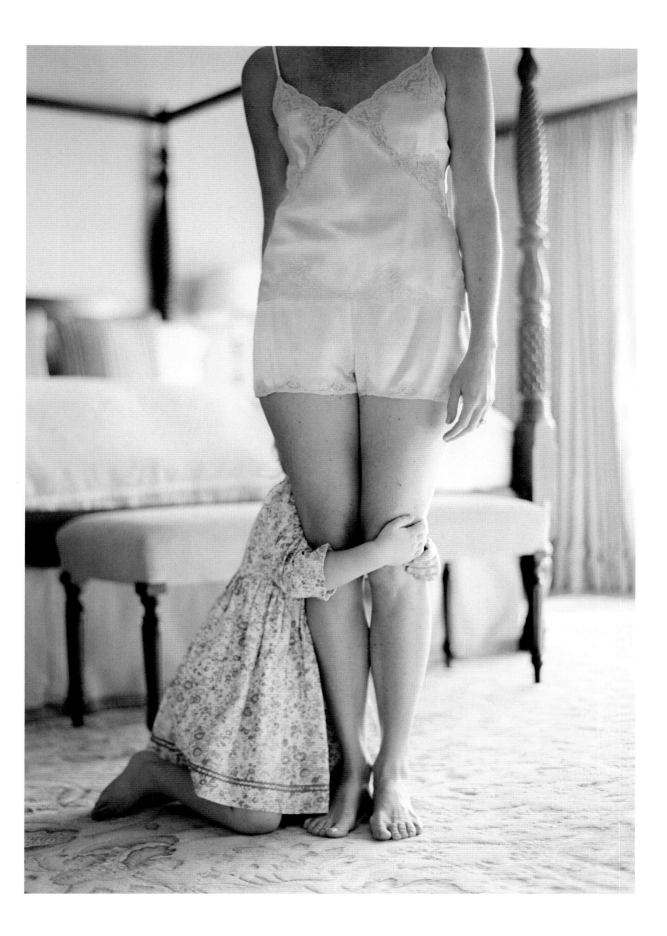

THE SILVER LINING

While we cannot protect all of the world's children from the big and little "lumps" (pun intended) of life, the manner in which the experience is handled lays the foundation for how children will handle the inevitable future "lumps" in the road. Children are wonderfully resilient and can survive a family's cancer diagnosis, treatment, and recovery.

We had two choices about how we were going to handle this breast cancer diagnosis: from a position of fear or from one of love, from a place of truth or from one of denial. We chose love and truth. As a result, our children mirrored our words, actions, and emotions. It was emotional. It was honest. It was exceptionally hard, but we were all in it together.

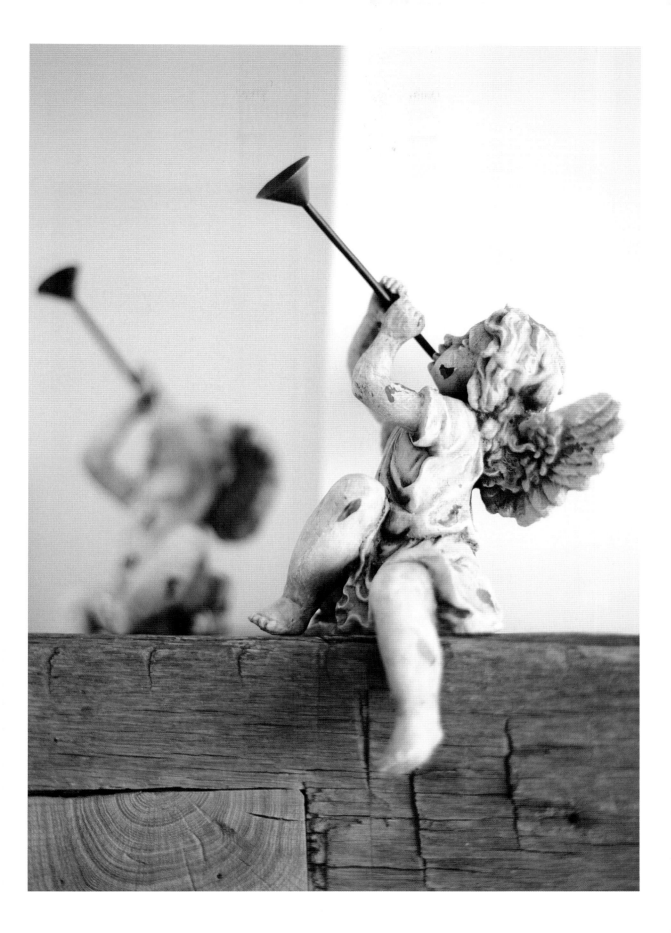

Stages of Development
What Is Typical. What They Know. What to Do.

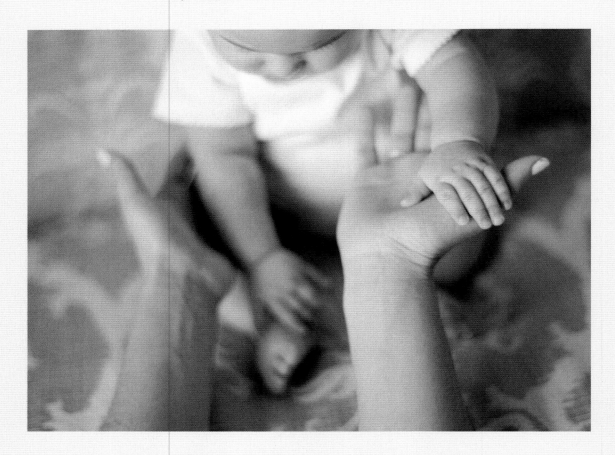

INFANTS (BIRTH TO TWELVE MONTHS)

WHAT IS TYPICAL: The first year of life is *busy*. Infants are focused on forming attachments, gaining control over motor skills, and developing an ability to regulate arousal and affect. They also develop language and object permanence (awareness that objects exist when out of sight). During infancy, memory also develops, as evidenced by their (dissatisfied!) reactions to separation from parents.

WHAT THEY UNDERSTAND: Think they have "no clue"? I'm sorry to burst that naive bubble, but infants are very aware when things go awry in a family. Though they have no cognitive concept of cancer, they are aware of tension, change in routine, unfamiliar environments, and most of all the separation from primary caregivers. These feelings have the potential to set off insecure patterns of attachment and/or hyperarousal (e.g., extended periods of crying) or withdrawal. Infants can also develop an irritable or "difficult" temperament combined with an inability to be soothed. This is how they demonstrate both the fact that they know something is going haywire and how they feel about it.

WHAT TO DO: Maintain a predictable environment with consistent caregivers. Please limit the number of caregivers so the infant doesn't become overwhelmed and confused. Provide comfort through touch, rocking, and by pacifiers (sucking) as well as with transitional objects, such as stuffed animals and/or and blankets.

TODDLERS (TWELVE MONTHS TO THREE YEARS)

WHAT IS TYPICAL: This period of development is all about exploration and discovery. Toddlers begin to recognize themselves as individuals, separate from their parents. During this period, there is an inherent push-pull when toddlers want to be with their parents but also want to do things on their own, e.g., "Me!" or "I do it!" Toddlers quickly learn the limits of their own bodies, which often results in frustration. Language skills blossom during this period, and toddlers are eager to express themselves using their new skills. Toddlers are focused on self-control and willpower. When they aren't in control or don't get their way is when tantrums can erupt.

WHAT THEY UNDERSTAND: Though toddlers cannot cognitively understand details about cancer, they too are aware when something is amiss in a family. They are most afraid of being separated from their parents and of medical procedures (e.g., surgery and "cutting") and treatment (e.g., chemotherapy and radiation) that they cannot understand.

WHAT TO DO: Maintain a consistent schedule. This point cannot be overstated. Provide information about cancer in simple, clear, and reassuring language. Communication using transitional objects such as dolls, puppets, or stuffed animals is helpful. Toddlers need to be reassured over and over and over again that they did nothing to cause the cancer, that it cannot be "caught," and that they will not be left alone. Engage a professional to help guide you through the process.

PRESCHOOL AGE (THREE TO SIX YEARS)

WHAT IS TYPICAL: To a preschooler, the world is a magical place, centered around the family. Preschoolers are fascinated with learning how things work. Everything that happens during this period stems from egocentricity. In other words, "It's all about *me*." They believe that all events happen in relation to them. Preschool children also believe that what happens around them happens because of them. Nice, right? In graduate school, I learned that "play is the work of children," which means that play is how children acquire information and grow: socially, physically, intellectually, and emotionally.

WHAT THEY UNDERSTAND: Preschool-age children understand the concept of cancer as an illness if explained in very literal, concrete terms. Concepts such as time and illness are not yet fully developed in the preschool period. Because magical thinking plays such a dominant role in preschoolers' lives, it extends to their thoughts about illness. Magical thinking enables them to think that they have the capacity to cause or fix a calamitous event, e.g., my daughter once told me: "I can get rid of your cancer by waving my magic wand." This philosophy can lead to feelings of guilt or anxiety because, in fact, they cannot actually cause or fix things. Preschoolers also use associative logic to connect seemingly unrelated things.

As a social worker, I was asked to work with Mia, a five-year-old who was having sleeping problems (insomnia and nightmares) after the death of her grandmother. As it turns out, shortly after the death of her grandmother, Mia overheard an adult conversation in which someone said, "Thank goodness Betty's death was so peaceful. When her time came, she just fell asleep and died." *Ding! Ding! Ding!* Mia thought that if she went to sleep that she could possibly die as well.

I'll also never forget Sarah, the four-year-old daughter of a man in hospice for whom I was caring. Despite the fact that her parents wanted to "protect" her from the pain of her father's death, the little girl knew. She said to me, "Daddy is dying but he doesn't want me to know."

WHAT TO DO: Describe cancer using simple, clear, and concise language. It is imperative to use the exact name of the disease and the associated body parts, e.g., "breast cancer." A preschooler needs constant reassurance that nothing he or she has done has caused the illness and that it is not a form of punishment. Repeatedly remind preschoolers that cancer is not contagious. They also need reassurance that they will not be left alone. It is superimportant to encourage feedback and provide the opportunity for children to ask questions and to share their emotions. After conversations, ask the child to summarize what she has heard. This provides the opportunity to clarify any misunderstanding. For the preschooler, a sense of security is derived from schedules and rules. I just can't overstate the need for maintaining a predictable, normal schedule and consistent limits.

While working as an adult hospice nurse, I cared for an elderly woman, a grandmother. Shortly after her death, I went to her home. When I walked in, her six-year-old grandson said to me, "Where are your wings?" My what? I asked. "Your *wings*. Mommy said that an angel was coming to take Granny to heaven." See what I mean about literal?

MIDDLE CHILDHOOD (SIX TO TWELVE YEARS)

WHAT IS TYPICAL: During middle childhood, children develop a sense of competence. They can now solve problems and understand rules and societal expectations of correct behavior. This is the beginning of abstract and logical thinking, but the tendency is still to be literal. As friendships develop, there is an increasing orientation toward peers. As children grow into middle childhood, they develop a sense of morality and the ability to decipher between right and wrong behavior. During middle childhood, a child takes pride in the ability to assume new responsibilities. By

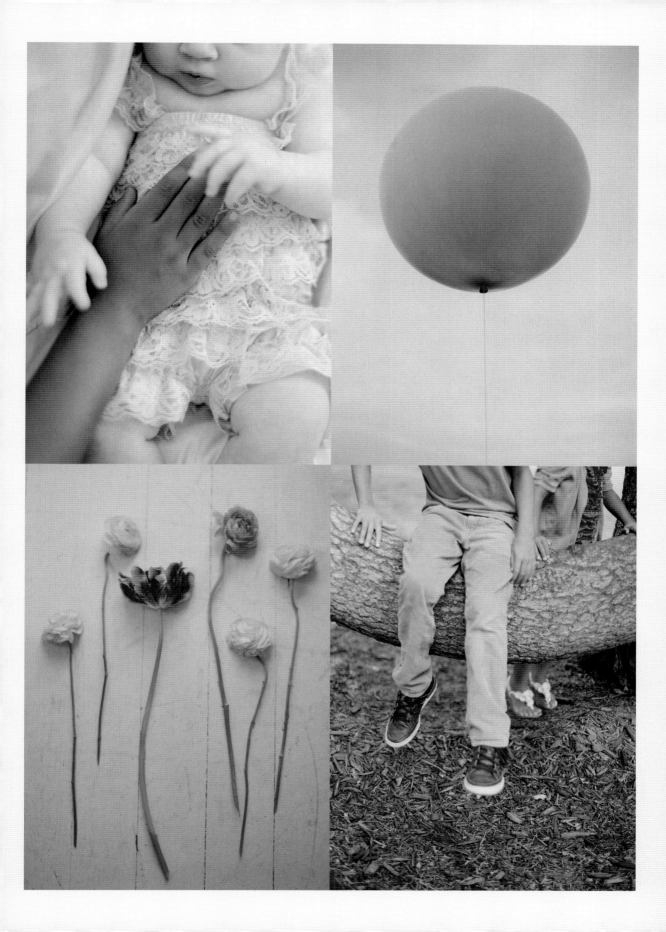

about ten, children have a clearer understanding of emotions and emotional nuances in themselves and others, e.g., recognizing when someone is sad or angry. Both short-term and long-term memory develops during middle childhood. There is a decline in egocentrism, which enables children to better understand and empathize with the needs of others.

WHAT THEY UNDERSTAND: Children in middle childhood have the capacity to understand and seek to learn the (very basic!) biologic processes of disease. They are, however, still in a transitional state and often find many words confusing, especially when some words have several meanings and connotations, for example, "soul."

I remember working with a nine-year-old who thought she heard her grandmother talking to her from a shoebox in a closet. In her mind, the "soul" of a person and the "sole" of a shoe were the same. Yup. I cannot overstress how important it is to *not* assume anything with children and to clarify everything.

Children in middle childhood are more practical in their understanding of and approach to treatment. They are more likely to understand that different treatments are necessary to treat cancer. Children at this age have the ability to listen attentively to all that is said but without always comprehending. They are often hesitant to ask questions or to admit not knowing something they think they should know.

They may have fears of abandonment and isolation. Often they think of illness as punishment for bad behavior. Though they are making a transition to a more adult understanding of the concept of illness, they will sometimes still have remnants of magical thinking and the "I caused it" syndrome.

WHAT TO DO: Children benefit from concrete specifics about cancer, but in simple terms. Use diagrams, pictures, and models for explanation because the thinking is concrete. Explain the meaning of cancer and any related words your child may hear. For example, an X-ray is "a picture of the inside of a body" or chemotherapy is "medicine to get rid of cancer." To avoid confusion and misunderstanding, it is helpful to ask the child to explain what she has heard from other people and, consequently, what she understands. Address any potential guilt issues (whether verbalized or not). Encourage children to become involved in family decision making when appropriate, e.g., what to have for dinner or initiating a play date. This makes them feel included.

Consistency and predictability are still very important; therefore, limit separation from family and friends as much as possible. Writing down and posting the weekly schedule can be helpful for children because it gives them the comfort of knowing what to expect in upcoming days. Encourage children to play because it enhances a child's feelings of control. Play also serves as a physical outlet for emotions and a temporary escape from the stress of a cancer diagnosis and treatment.

If possible, ask children if they would like to meet your doctor or see how the doctors and nurses are going to care for you. Though, be sure to ask your doctor first!

When Lalee turned six, I asked whether she would like to meet my doctor. She responded with an enthusiastic "*Yes!*" She wrote a lot of questions prior to the meeting (which took place during a scheduled appointment). Not all children want to participate in such a way, however. Always and in all ways, it is important to respect their wishes.

ADOLESCENTS (TWELVE YEARS AND OLDER)

WHAT IS TYPICAL: Adolescence is a period of immense and often intense emotional and physical growth. Their bodies (and often moods!) change right before our eyes. Though most adolescents still have respect for their parents and other authority figures, this is the time when being with peers is much more enticing than being with family. In fact, peers become the barometer for assessing normalcy.

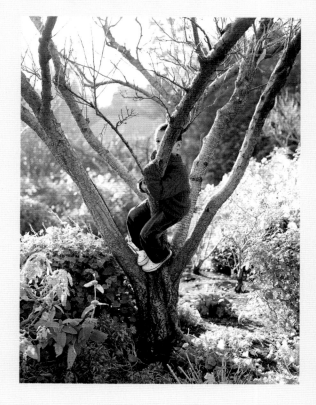

Teens tend to be narcissistic and often engage in risk-taking behaviors (which makes me want to bubble wrap Lalee!). Part of their identity development comes from testing limits and boundaries (more bubble wrap, please!). Adolescents are aware of societal expectations— though they may not agree with them—and begin to think about and plan for the future.

WHAT THEY UNDERSTAND: Adolescents are able to understand the biological and psychological aspects of cancer. Cognitively, they have the ability to understand the complex, scientific aspects of cancer and often want to learn details about the disease and treatment options. They may also become philosophical and ask questions such as, "What is the meaning of cancer?"

It is typical for them to wonder how the cancer will affect their life, e.g., "Will Mom still make dinner every night?" or "Who will drive me to soccer practice?" or even "I'm so embarrassed that my Mom is bald."

Additionally, they also want to know what their responsibilities will be, such as cleaning, cooking, and/or caring for other children in the family. Added responsibility commonly results in feelings of resentment and anger, which can then lead to fear and guilt.

Existentially, adolescents have a new awareness of life's vulnerability. All of a sudden, they become aware of their own mortality by acknowledging that life is transient and that nobody lives forever. See what I mean about big changes?!?

WHAT TO DO: Because teenagers have the capacity to understand the basic facts about a diagnosis and treatment plan, talk openly and candidly with them. Ask them how much they already know about cancer (i.e., to potentially eliminate misconceptions) and then ask how much they want to know. Allow them to choose not to know every detail.

It's important to remember that even though a teenager has the capacity to understand a disease diagnosis and treatment, adults should not overestimate this capacity. In other words, they may act like they know more than they actually do. To ensure clarity and avoid confusion and misunderstanding, ask them to repeat what they heard in the discussion(s). Also,

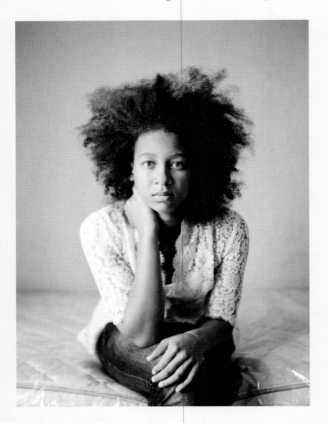

because so many adolescents have access to the Internet, ask them to avoid doing independent research, because the findings are often inaccurate and have the potential to exacerbate confusion and fear. Instead, I recommend going online together (to sites recommended by a health care professional) to discuss what specifically interests them.

When adolescents are confronted with illness in the family, they need sensitive guidance and help processing emotions. Often, the person best able to help is not in the family. Please don't take this personally. It really isn't about you. The most helpful person could actually be a teacher, counselor, coach, or neighbor. The most important thing is to identify who that person is and to respect the adolescent's privacy and opinions by not prying or being judgmental.

It is important to encourage adolescents to maintain their lives as much as possible. However, when they help pick up the slack in a family by cleaning, cooking, or even running errands, acknowledging how hard the situation is will go a long way in building a familial bond.

Zach, an adolescent boy with whom I worked, overheard (through a wall!) that his mother had stage II cancer. He didn't know how many stages of cancer existed and assumed, because she wouldn't talk about it, that hers was the worst and that she was inevitably going to die. The reality, however, was that his mother's cancer, though requiring challenging treatment, was very treatable. His mother, bless her heart, didn't know how to talk with her son and therefore just didn't. The bottom line is this: adolescents have the capacity to understand and interest in knowing the big picture. Trust and include them in the process.

Questions Children Ask

In my professional—and now personal—experiences, I have found that children often wonder—either aloud or silently—these five questions. I highly recommend bringing these questions up with children, whether they articulate them or not. Another helpful hint: when answering a child's question, don't give rambling answers. In other words, answer the question that is asked and no more. Too much information can be overwhelming and can interfere with his or her ability to process.

WHAT IS CANCER? Begin with a very simple explanation: *Our bodies, including our breasts, are made up of cells. Cells are tiny. We can't see them but they are what make our bodies work. Cancer cells don't work or act like normal cells. They are not nice and don't treat other cells nicely. Cancer cells grow very fast and cause a person's body to not work correctly.*

For some children, this amount of information is all they can handle at one time. This is perfectly normal. This is, after all, an incredibly intense situation. Going slower is better, and delivering small amounts of information at a time is optimal. As we always say in our home, "Slow and steady wins the race."

DID I CAUSE THE CANCER? This question arises directly from magical thinking. All too often, children as young as age three have the potential to assume that they have played some hand in causing the cancer, for example: "Because I was mad at Mommy, she got cancer." This is the question that children often keep to themselves, because they feel responsibility and guilt for a diagnosis. This is the reason that adults have to address this issue head-on and assuage any misconceptions. Before she had the opportunity to wonder, we told Lalee that no one caused the cancer. It wasn't Mommy's fault. It wasn't Daddy's fault. It wasn't Lalee's fault.

IS IT CONTAGIOUS? Just because we adults know that cancer is not contagious does not mean that children know it. Children understand that colds are contagious, so it is easy, especially for younger children, to use associative logic to connect cancer with a cold. After all, they both begin with the letter C. Be sure to explain that cancer is not in any way, shape, or form contagious.

WHO WILL TAKE CARE OF ME WHILE MOMMY IS SICK? Children are afraid of being left alone. They need to be assured that someone they know—father, other family member, friend, or neighbor—will be there to take care of them during treatment. Consistency of routine and of caregiver is of utmost importance because they equate to security. During my treatment, my husband and I assembled "Team Lalee" to lovingly care for her.

ARE YOU GOING TO DIE? Inevitably, the subject of death will come up. People do die from breast cancer. When this topic arises, as difficult as it may be, parents need to be completely open to answer questions honestly, without evasion or embarrassment. If you say that you aren't going to die and then you do, not only are you dead, but you are also a liar. I'm just saying. It's the truth.

To learn more, I highly recommend these two books: *When a Parent Has Cancer* by Dr. Wendy Schlessel Harpham and *How to Help Children Through a Parent's Serious Illness* by Kathleen McCue.

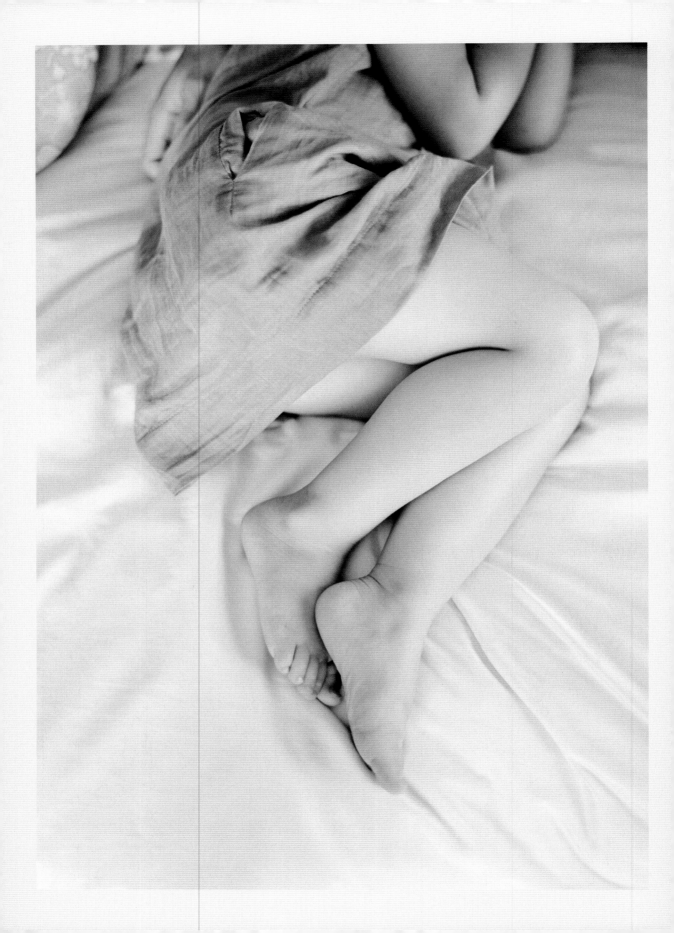

Support & Suggestions for Talking with Children

PREPARE for the conversation by writing down talking points and rehearsing what you are going to say. Seriously. It really helped me!

PLAN where and when you will have the conversation, ideally when the children are most awake and capable of focusing. We had our conversation in the morning.

BE AT EYE LEVEL WITH A CHILD. This may sound silly, but it is important that children not feel spoken down to. Lalee sat on my lap, facing me.

PROVIDE A "WARNING SHOT" or an introductory sentence before delivering potentially alarming news, for example: "I have some important and sad news to tell you."

JUST DO IT. Take a deep breath and tell them. Even though it is hard, it will be much worse (yes, it can get worse!) if they overhear the news from someone else.

USE DEVELOPMENTALLY APPROPRIATE LANGUAGE. Ask for professional guidance from a social worker, nurse, or counselor. You could even have someone with you to help describe the cancer in detail. Asking for help and support is a Silver Lining.

SPEAK IN A CLEAR, CALM, UNHURRIED, AND CONFIDENT VOICE. Be specific and use simple words and short sentences. I counted to three between points to give time for Lalee to respond.

BEGIN WITH BASIC INFORMATION, and let the child's questions direct the conversation.

ENCOURAGE FEEDBACK AND QUESTIONS. Answer questions honestly. If you don't know the answer, let them know that you will find out and get back to them.

PREPARE FOR MULTIPLE CONVERSATIONS, over time. Remember: this is a marathon, not a sprint. Children can digest only so much at a time. Let them process in bits and pieces.

USE A VARIETY OF COMMUNICATION TECHNIQUES to encourage dialogue and expression, such as books, games, art, music, and movies.

MODEL HEALTHY COPING MECHANISMS and share emotions. Tell them what you feel (e.g., sad and confused), but reassure them that you will get through it together.

COMMUNICATE WITH TEACHERS AND SCHOOL COUNSELORS so that they can help support children at school.

CHAPTER III

Lost & Found
Navigating the Surgical Experience

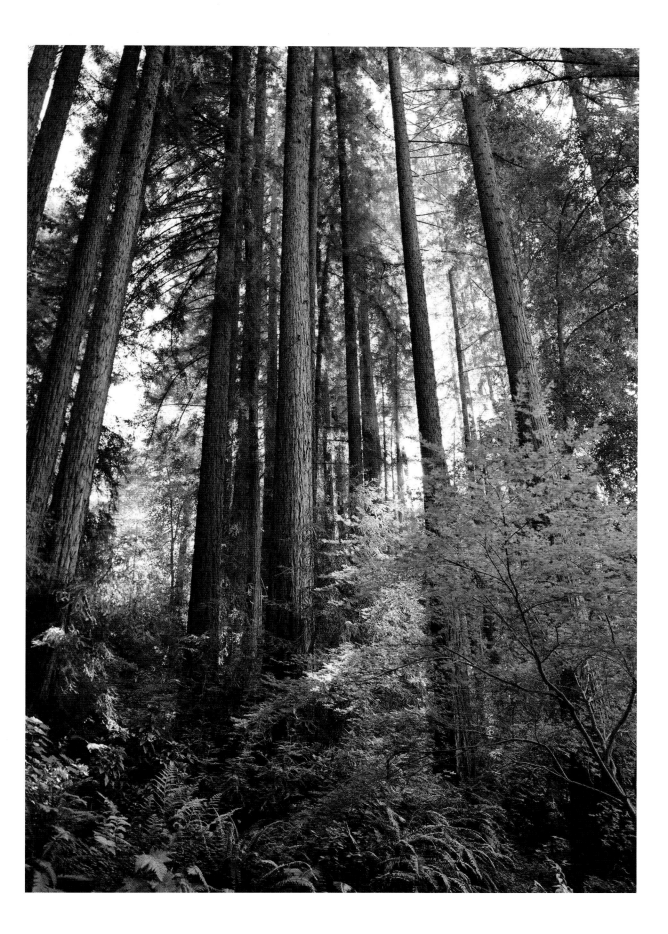

With an official diagnosis of breast cancer, I felt lost, as if I were standing in the middle of a dense, tangled, cobweb-filled forest, one in which I had never been. I was unsure which way to turn or how to proceed.

As a nurse and social worker, I had the unique perspective of having seen patients in this exact same wretchedly frightening and confusing place. My clinical experience enabled me to visualize a vista from which I was able to create the road map out of the haze. I put my professional hat on and pondered, "How would I handle this situation if I were counseling a patient?" And, more personally, "What would I say to a newly diagnosed friend? And then myself!?" Here are four tips that really helped me:

1. "Breathe." It sounds easy, I know, but when you hear the words "You have cancer," breathing actually takes focused effort.

2. Though the diagnosis feels like an emergency, it's not. You have time to understand the meaning and process the emotions of your diagnosis. Even if it feels as though your doctor seems to know exactly what to do before you can get your bearings, do *not* feel pressured to make a quick, on-the-spot decision about treatment.

3. Learn everything you can about your diagnosis and treatment options. One big misconception is that doctors develop a patient's plan of care on their own. No, no, no. Patients have a real responsibility to be fully engaged in the development (and revision) of a plan of care.

4. Build a team of caregivers and advisers, both personal (friends) as well as professional (health care providers). You know that phrase "It takes a village"? Well, it definitely takes a village to get through breast cancer.

Boy, did that help me gain the perspective that I desperately needed.

After a weekend of diagnosis digestion and announcement making, my husband and I had an information-gathering week in order to fully understand the diagnosis and make decisions about the course of my treatment. One Silver Lining in this whole mess was that my husband and I are good—really good—planners and expeditious decision makers.

LIFELINE

Working in health care has taught me that it is imperative for people to be consumer driven. Personally, this translated into interviewing & hiring the people with whom I felt the most comfortable & confident.

INTERVIEWING

Even though you are thrust into an unknown world, full of medical jargon and white coats, *you* are still empowered to interview and hire the team of people who will care for you. During this interviewing and hiring process, it is important to seek (and find!) chemistry with the people who will care for you. In addition to education, training, and experience, the things that were important to me included having my questions fully answered to my satisfaction in an unrushed, focused manner. I don't like waiting in general, but with breast cancer, any delay turned on my grumpy button. So a punctual office was very important to me. I also paid close attention to how the physicians treated their staff. I noticed whether they were abrupt and rude or kind and respectful. You can guess in which direction I went.

Now, I know there are the unsavory golden handcuffs of insurance with which we all must contend. The reality is that most insurance programs and/or medical offices dictate that information. However, it doesn't cost a thing to gather information, which is what we did.

My husband and I met with the following doctors:

- two surgical oncologists (surgeons who specialize in breast cancer)
- three medical oncologists (doctors who specialize in treating cancer with chemotherapy)
- two radiation oncologists (doctors who specialize in radiation of cancer)
- two plastic surgeons (doctors who specialize in reconstruction after a mastectomy)
- one palliative care physician (doctor who specializes in pain management)

Whoa. Whoa. Whoa. Are you wondering, "Why palliative care?" Most people hear the phrase "palliative care" and think "Buy the plot . . . she must be dying." We met with a palliative care physician *not* because I was dying but because palliative care provides expertise in pain and symptom management.

As a nurse and now patient, I am all too familiar with the fact that surgeons and oncologists, despite inflicting a great amount of pain on their patients, are not experts in pain management. Quite ironic, if you ask me. But it's the truth. The Silver Lining is that there is a specialty focused on relieving pain and symptoms and it's called . . . *palliative care*!

> **LIFELINE**
>
> *Be sure to ask for a palliative care consultation when building your team of care. It's great pain & symptom management insurance!*

Anyway, I obviously knew that I wanted palliative care as part of my team in the event that I had any unique pain or symptom issues that required specialized treatment. Trust me, there is always the potential for unique circumstances.

Before each of my doctor appointments, my husband and I prepared a list of questions. Why? Well, under the duress of a world-rocking diagnosis, it is easy, so easy, to forget what you want to ask at the precise moment that you want to ask it. My list included clarifying questions about my diagnosis as well as inquiries into treatment options.

The information-gathering week also included a series of tests, beginning with a PET scan to analyze what was going on with the lesions in my left breast and an enlarged lymph node. Did I forget to mention that lymph node? Sorry. The stress of a breast cancer diagnosis made me a little forgetful. An enlarged lymph node jumped out on the original MRI and warranted further investigation.

My PET scan was inconclusive, meaning that it was not possible to determine whether the tumors in the left breast were cancerous or not. I was told that in all likelihood, one, if not all, of the tumors was either cancerous or precancerous. The only way to tell for sure was with an MRI-guided breast biopsy. In other words, the only way to get a sample of the tissue from the tumor was to have an MRI machine guide the physician (and a very long needle) into the tumor. If I decided, however, to go straightaway with the double mastectomy, that test would not be needed. *Hmmm.*

> **LIFELINE**
>
> *Go through your list of questions prior to the meeting to make sure that you have included everything you want to ask. Make two copies of the list to take with you to your appointment, one for the person going with you & one for your physician.*

The truth is that I had already decided to do a double mastectomy. There was no question in my mind. Having confirmed cancer in the right breast and suspicious tissue in the left breast made me feel pretty doggone confident that if I didn't have a double mastectomy, I would spend an inordinate amount of time worrying and waiting for the other shoe, I mean diagnosis, to drop.

I didn't want to live every day with a very real worry that the precancerous tumors could turn into cancer. It was just common sense, to me, to remove both breasts at the same time. It was my decision and my doctors and family concurred.

In terms of timing, I was inclined to follow the lead of my BFF, LiFT, who had a double mastectomy and reconstruction during the same surgery. After all, I spent the first two nights in the hospital with her after her surgery (because that's what nurse BFFs do for each other!), and though it was grueling, one of the first things she said after surgery was, "I'm glad I did it all at one time."

Now, I'm all about making the right decision, at the right time, for the right reason. In fact, it is a philosophy that I try to live my everyday life by and this situation was no different. In my decision-making process, I didn't want to jeopardize any treatment options just because I wanted to consolidate the double mastectomy and reconstruction surgeries. I kept my mind open but hoped that doing the double mastectomy and reconstruction simultaneously was a viable option.

My first meeting with a surgical oncologist (breast cancer surgeon) resulted in a big, fat bummer when he said, "Absolutely not. I will not do a mastectomy and reconstruction simultaneously. You *must* wait at least six months before I will do reconstruction."

"Why?" I asked.

"Because radiation will destroy the newly reconstructed tissue," the surgeon said.

"I thought you said you didn't yet know if I'd need radiation," I said.

"You probably will," he said.

Really? I was hoping to live in a state of denial for just a teensy bit longer.

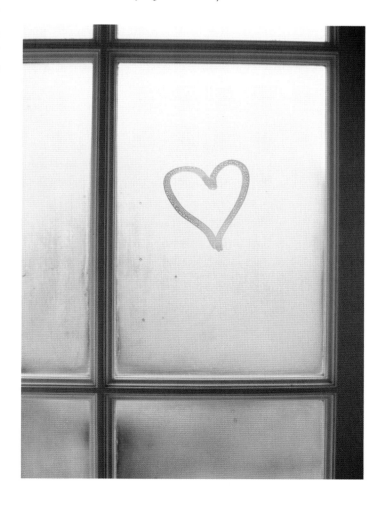

In the meantime, I was referred to another surgical oncologist and plastic surgeon team in Los Angeles. This meeting produced a polar opposite response when the new surgeons told my husband and me, "Absolutely, we can do a double mastectomy and reconstruction at the same time. This makes perfect sense and is a completely reasonable option." This made me want to do a happy dance!

Working with this team felt right, which leads me back to the subject of intuition. I am a firm believer in intuition. In fact, intuition played a wonderfully inspiring and significant role in my entire process.

There was an incredible synchronicity with this physician team and seamlessness to the decision-making process. In fact, *not* doing reconstruction was not given as a viable option. "It is better," we were told, "to do the reconstruction simultaneously because of the fresh tissue, superior aesthetic, and skin preservation."

Considering the previous meeting with the plastic surgeon who said that radiation would destroy the new tissue, I asked about the impact of radiation, postreconstruction (whether I had to have it was yet to be decided). My newly hired (yes, I pretty much hired him on the spot!) plastic surgeon told me that radiation would render the outcome less desirable and that I would have radiation effects that I would not like; however, doing reconstruction at the time of the double mastectomy was still the much better choice.

The surgeon went on to say that because I was thin and had small breasts, the best surgical option for me would be a staged implant reconstruction approach. In stage one (which takes place during the first surgery), I would have a modified radical mastectomy in which both breasts, including the skin, breast tissue, areolae, nipples, as well as most lymph nodes under the arms, would be removed. In this type of mastectomy, the lining over the pectoralis major muscle would be removed, but the pectoralis major muscle itself would be preserved.

During the surgery, "expanders" would be placed on the chest wall under the pectoralis major muscle for a period of time (anywhere from six to nine months for me, postradiation). A tissue expander is a temporary device that is placed on the chest wall under the pectoralis major muscle. The purpose of the expander is to create a soft pocket into which the implant would eventually go. The next stage would be replacing the expanders with implants (yes, this meant two surgeries), but the Silver Lining was that the second surgery and recovery time would be shorter than other reconstruction options (described at the end of this chapter).

LIFELINE

During your discussion, ask your surgeons to show you an illustration of what the mastectomy & reconstruction options look like. Having the visual helps the verbal explanation sink in!

Given my initial pathology results (showing that I had a more aggressive, invasive type of breast cancer), my only option was to have a modified radical double mastectomy. At the end of that meeting, the doctors and I even coordinated calendars and secured a date (ten days later) for the double mastectomy and reconstruction. Prior to my leaving, my newly hired surgeons gave me some preoperative instructions and sent me on my way, encouraging me to rest and relax (*ha!*) before surgery.

There was a great comfort in solidifying a plan. It felt as if I were moving forward.

WAITING AND PLANNING

It felt so strange to live ten days knowing that I had cancer in my body. I really wanted it *out-out-out*. But I had to wait. I found myself looking at my breasts and thinking, "Really, Girls? How did we get so off course? I thought we had a good thing going on. You fed my baby girl. You look pretty good in a bathing suit. Now you're going to *leave*?"

It was a very long ten days, but during that period, knowing that I was going to be out of commission for at least a few weeks, I had a lot to do, including interviewing oncologists, talking with our children, communicating with other family members and friends about the plan of care, and generally getting my life and my family's life in order before surgery.

At the top of the list was organizing our household. I knew that if my family was well cared for, then I would be better positioned to focus on healing. For the record, I run a fairly tight and organized ship. I knew, however, that I would not be doing any ship running for at least several weeks postsurgery. I wouldn't even be able to lift my arms high enough to get a glass from the flipping cabinet. Seriously. Oh, and no driving for several weeks either. So, I had to take a deep breath and actually bring myself to ask people for *help*. Oh, dear heavens, was that ever hard for me. The Silver Lining was that I had a slew of people who were eagerly waiting for marching orders, looking for things to do.

So, I made a list of all of the household fundamentals that I would need assistance with, such as postsurgery food delivery, preschool pickup and dropoff, and shopping, and (still begrudgingly) I asked for *help*. Though being vulnerable and receiving assistance went against every fiber of my being, I knew that it was necessary and the right thing to do.

After our household plan was in place, I came to the realization that the four-month work sabbatical that I had taken to move to Santa Barbara would now have to

> **LIFELINE**
>
> *Before treatments begin, make a list of all of your household needs & then ask family & friends for assistance.*

be extended. The Silver Lining was that I was in a very fortunate position to be able to take time off from my career. The health care field provides a great opportunity to leave and return as life circumstances ebb and flow, so I knew that when I was done with treatment, I could go back.

Many of my patients, however, are not so fortunate. The Silver Lining for them is that most companies are flexible and supportive when a person is stricken with breast cancer, or any kind of cancer for that matter. And if the company's not, there's a special place in h–e–double hockey sticks for them.

The week before surgery, my husband and I met with three oncologists regarding decisions that had to be made about my treatment after surgery. Everyone basically said the same thing: "Because you are so young and because you have multiple tumors, you will probably have to have chemotherapy and radiation after surgery." Fan-flippin'-tastic. When I asked two of the preliminary oncologists whom they recommended for palliative care, they gasped and said, "You don't neeeeeed palliative care! You're not dyyyyying!" I clearly knew that they were not going to be my oncologists, but I did take the opportunity to educate them about the fact that I wanted palliative care for pain management.

It was the third oncologist who, before I could even ask for a palliative care referral, said, "I have all of my patients meet with palliative care before treatment." I beamed and said, "You're hired." Then he went on to say, "I recommend that you get a second opinion to corroborate your treatment plan." I thought to myself, "Now, *this* is a great doctor!"

During the week before my surgery, we also got my insurance all figured out. It was the last thing in the world that I wanted to think about, but it was a necessity, considering my hospital bill alone would be well over a hundred thousand dollars! Fortunately, my husband is the person in our family who handles our insurance, but getting the insurance ducks in a row was a joint effort, considering the magnitude of logistics involved.

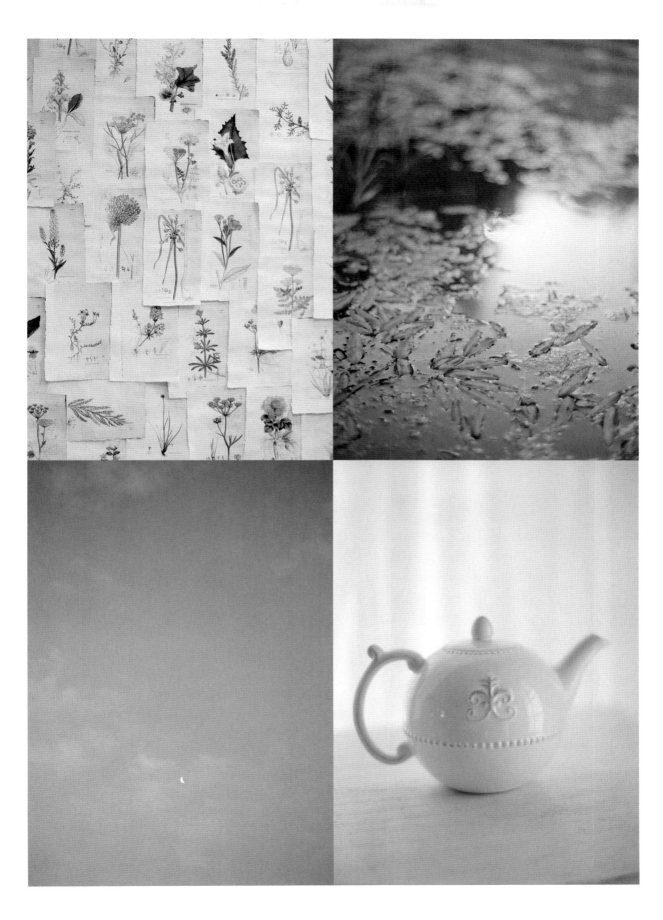

There wasn't a day that I didn't express gratitude for my insurance. As a nurse and social worker, I have worked with a multitude of people who were under- or un-insured. It was often heartbreaking to walk into patients' homes and see piles of paperwork and the reflection of worry on their faces. I mean, really, not only were they contending with the devastation of a diagnosis combined with outrageously expensive treatments, but they were also swimming in a sea of paperwork and debt.

Though it is still overwhelming, there are a few Silver Linings to help. CancerCare (cancercare.org) and the Patient Advocate Foundation (copays.org) are terrific organizations that have financial assistance programs and resources. Additionally, denials can be contested. I remember a bill for twenty-seven thousand dollars that my insurance company refused to pay (it gives me palpitations even thinking about it). However, we contested it and won. When in doubt, call your insurance company and learn what benefits you have and what will be covered.

Three days before surgery, I went for some routine tests, including a blood test, urinalysis, and electrocardiogram (EKG). These tests assess whether your body is ready (or as ready as it can be) for the surgery.

Two days before surgery, I packed. After all, I wanted to be strategic and thoughtful about what I took to the hospital. Whenever I pack the night before I go somewhere, I *always* forget something. I really didn't want to be at the hospital wishing for this or that. Fortunately, with the help of my LiFT, I compiled a winning list that ensured that I had everything I needed.

The day before surgery, I had three preregistration phone calls covering everything from insurance questions to allergies to whether I was taking any drugs (including herbal supplements). I understood the need to acquire this information for my ever-growing medical chart. What I didn't understand was the need to have three phone calls, all of which asked or told me the exact same information. My patience as a patient was pushed to a near breaking point. Was no one listening the first or even the second time? By the third phone call, I asked to speak to a supervisor (always a good idea!) to ensure that I would not have to go through the rigmarole again.

The Silver Lining of the day before the

LIFELINE

Ask for help with insurance & bills. Fees can be discounted & negotiated. Don't do it alone!

LIFELINE

Make a comprehensive list (use mine as an example; see page 92) of everything that you need to pack before going to the hospital. As you pack, check the items off the list to ensure that you remember everything.

surgery was that my dearest girlfriend, LiFT, flew in to be with me. She took a week out of her very full life to be my personal nurse advocate in the hospital and to get my postsurgical self home. Yes, this was the same friend who had breast cancer a year and a half before my diagnosis. It sounds crazy, right? I mean two best friends from nursing school who both get breast cancer within a year and a half. Who could have imagined such a thing? I know that we certainly couldn't have.

I was overwhelmed by her gesture of love. The moment she arrived, she said, "We really need to start meeting at spas rather than in hospitals." No kidding. She is also the friend who told me "We. Know. How. To. Do. This.," which was a guiding Silver Lining throughout my treatment.

The night before surgery, we went to a fancy-schmancy fashion party in Los Angeles. It was much better than anxiously pacing around my hotel room . . . waiting. I was so glad I went because it gave me perspective; I knew that although at the same time the next night, I would still be under sedation after having my breasts removed, life would go on.

Between my diagnosis and surgery, a friend who had had a double mastectomy recommended that I take a photo of my breasts so that I could remember them. *Geesh,* writing that even seems weird. However, the friend who made the recommendation is a smartie. She said, "You were born with your breasts and have had them for thirty-nine years. They fed your daughter and helped give her life. You'll want a memory."

So, after showering and washing myself with the required, unchic antibacterial soap and before going to sleep, I put on a robe and looked (and felt) a little haggard. My husband said, "Let's take the photo." Feeling exceptionally unsexy and anxious, I pulled my robe down and he took two photos, one with my face and breasts and one with just my breasts. Not exactly a Richard Avedon image, but I trusted my girlfriend who promised me that I would be glad I did. She was right.

> ## LIFELINE
>
> *If you are taking any medication or are allergic to any medication, the surgeon & the anesthesiologist must be informed. Also let your surgeon & anesthesiologist know whether you are taking any herbal supplements because some can increase a person's risk of bleeding & therefore must be discontinued before surgery.*

> ## LIFELINE
>
> *Before a mastectomy, take a photograph of your breasts. Even if you don't intend to look at it, just take it. One day, someday, you may be really glad that you did. I know I am.*

SURGERY

The moment that the clock struck midnight (yes, I should have been asleep!) officially began the day of my surgery. I was no longer able to eat or drink anything prior to the procedure (no matter how hungry or thirsty I was). This is standard protocol to ensure that your stomach is completely empty during surgery. There's something suffocating about being told that you "can't" do something, especially something as natural and normal as eating or drinking.

Despite having three hospital preregistration phone calls during which I was asked the same questions and given the same instructions ("What is your insurance number?" "Are you on any medications?" "Do you take supplements?" "Who will be taking you home from the hospital?" "Wear comfortable clothes," "Don't bring anything valuable," etc.) *and* arriving at five in the morning as we were told, we sat on the floor (because the waiting room was full and there were no more empty chairs) for an hour and a half. It was not exactly a presurgical mood enhancer, if you know what I mean.

At a little after seven o'clock I was finally called back to the surgical preparation area. You would have thought that I had done something very wrong by the way the doctors and nurses were speaking in punitive tones and frenetically hustling and bustling around me. When I asked whether there was a problem, my nurse said, "Your surgery is supposed to start *now*." As politely as I could, I told her that I had been sitting (on the floor, no less!) behind (and I pointed to it) *that door,* a mere fifty yards away.

Right before surgery, there was actually *a lot* to do, beginning with removing all jewelry and clothes and changing into yet another unattractive hospital gown. Next, I had a physical examination and interview by the anesthesiologist. During our conversation, we discussed the fact that morphine doesn't work for my pain management and that I wanted to have Dilaudid (a much stronger form of intravenous pain medicine). He promised that he would order Dilaudid for my PCA machine.

A patient-controlled analgesia (PCA) is a method of pain control that gives the patient the power to control his or her pain. In a PCA, a computerized pump—called the patient-controlled analgesia pump—that contains a syringe of pain medicine prescribed by a doctor is connected directly to a patient's intravenous (IV) line. Pain medicine is delivered continously and/or the patient pushes a button to receive pain medicine when needed.

By the way, are you wondering how I knew what pain medication I wanted? Well, two years prior to this breast cancer nonsense, I had spinal meningitis. Yep. However, over the course of four spinal taps, I had a variety of different pain management medications to get pain relief. Therefore, I knew that Dilaudid was the right pain medication for me.

After the anesthesiologist left, my oncology breast surgeon and plastic surgeon

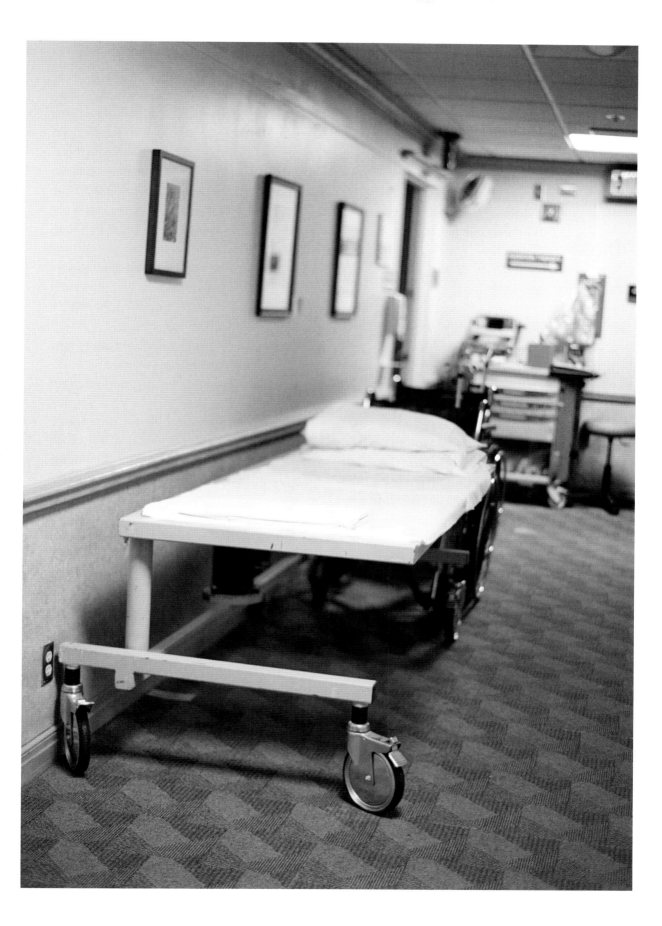

came in so that they could outline the procedure—literally. They used black Sharpie markers to tattoo a connect-the-dots-esque drawing on my chest to remind them what to do in surgery. Go ahead and laugh, because the memory of them drawing on my breasts with a Sharpie deserves a chuckle.

Next, the nurse asked me a seemingly unending list of questions: "What is your insurance number?" "Are you taking any medications?" "Do you take supplements?" "Have you eaten or had anything to drink since midnight?" "Who will be bringing you home from the hospital?" Yes, these were the same questions that had been asked and answered on at least five other occasions over the past week. Yes, it was annoying. However, the nurse in me acknowledged how necessary it was to prevent mistakes from being made. For a patient, though, it was really, truly, and utterly aggravating!

> ## LIFELINE
> *Though the IV may hurt going in, after insertion, it should no longer hurt. If it does, be sure to let your nurse know.*

Then the nurse started an IV line in my arm, through which a lovely sedative (Versed) was administered. Within minutes, the medication helped me relax.

It wasn't until I was waiting for the surgery, lying naked (except for a short hospital gown) on the gurney, tattooed, IV in my arm, that it really hit me that I was having my breasts removed (not that I had cancer, but that I was having my breasts *removed*). I wasn't sad or scared. Not because I was brave. I wasn't—or didn't feel—brave at all. Rather, it was more like, "Whoa. This is really happening. I'm having my *breasts removed*."

When my nurse said, "It's time to go," I became fairly emotional (cue the tears). Saying good-bye to my husband was one of the hardest things I've ever done in my life. The look on his face was heartbreaking.

Being rolled into surgery and transferred onto the operating table (for some reason I thought that I would have been asleep by now, but no, I was *wide* awake) was in and of itself a unique experience. Of course my inner nurse was fascinated by the gazillions of gadgets and gizmos being prepped by the surgical nurses. There were *soooooo* many.

Before I could really start to count the surgical instruments, my anesthesiologist told me that he was going to put some medication in my IV to make me go to sleep. "How quickly?" I asked. "Before you can count to ten," he said. "One . . . two . . . zzzzzzz . . . ," I think I said.

During the surgery, my husband wrote on the blog:

> *Reality was very strong this morning for us both. That feeling you get when you wake up and there is the feeling of dread. I watched her get prepared for surgery. It was all I could do to keep from*

crying. The doctors wrote on her chest what exactly was supposed to be removed. They gave her a little Versed for her to help her relax. They don't offer that to the husband. I'll put that on my comment card along with the coffee dearth at 5am. It's the worst feeling to see a loved one rolled away for surgery. Expecting up to 7 hours of surgery. I'll be waiting in the cafeteria with her best friend. Coffee, magazines, iPad and fear.

First part of surgery complete, about 2 ½ hours left to go for the reconstruction part. The surgeon said he did need to take some lymph nodes on the right side. Hope to get the complete pathology back by Friday. More when we know.

She came out of surgery approximately five hours after going in. She was in the recovery room for a couple hours and then transferred to a hospital room. Next key information needed is the pathology report, which will inform chemotherapy and radiation decisions. Hope to take her home in three or four days. Continued thanks for the prayers and good wishes.

Just saw her for the first time, what a relief, she's groggy from the drugs and asked for ice chips, but it's her, with her beautiful smile, I love her so much.

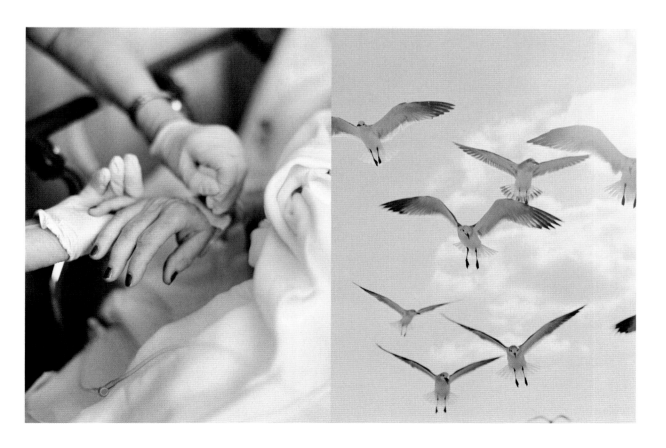

RECOVERY, SORT OF

I remembered nothing about recovery or room transfer. Instead, I woke up in a pitch-black room, nearly glued to the ceiling with pain. Pain the likes of which I had never experienced before, ever. My first thought was, "Something is really *wrong*. It shouldn't hurt this *much*." Through my tears, I woke up LiFT, who was sleeping next to me. I could barely talk. Thankfully, she assessed the situation immediately and went into action.

First, she looked at my PCA. She read the number and said, "This can't be right." Then she called the nurse into the room and insisted on knowing how much pain medicine I had received. The nurse was silent for a long time and then said, "None."

Yes, you read that correctly. After having had both breasts removed and reconstructed, now twelve hours after the surgery, I had had absolutely *no* pain medication. "Are you flipping kidding me?" (though I think that she may have used a different "f" word), I heard LiFT say . . . followed closely with, "Get the doctor on the phone *now*."

How on earth was this possible? you might wonder. Well, after I came to my senses, I wondered the exact same thing, especially because I had taken every single precaution to ensure proper pain management. In addition to talking with the anesthesiologist, I discussed the importance—the *priority*—of pain management post-amputation and reconstruction with every nurse and physician I met. "Nurses on the floor are trained in pain management," I was told by one physician. "*No, they are not,*" I said firmly. "I *know* about inadequate pain management training because this used to be my job, which is why I am telling you exactly what I want and when," I said.

As it turns out, I was given morphine after surgery (remember that I asked for Dilaudid because I knew that morphine didn't work for me?). In the recovery room, my husband noticed this mistake and told the nurses that I wanted the Dilaudid. "Oh, that's right. We will change it," they said. Well, they did indeed change it, but after they put the cartridge of Dilaudid in the pump, they forgot to turn it *on*. Uh-huh. Let that sink in for a sec. Or don't.

Are you wondering why I am so obsessed with pain management? Well, because pain is *bad. Bad. Bad.* Pain interrupts sleep. Pain decreases mobility. Pain decreases endurance and energy. Pain strains resources by producing such symptoms as fatigue, depression, and constipation. Pain can also impair the immune response and your subsequent ability to get *better*. Unrelieved pain can cause permanent damage to the nervous system. Get it? Pain is *bad, really bad.*

Virtually nothing positive can resume (relationships, activities of daily living, thinking, etc.) until physical pain is managed. Think about it this

---

LIFELINE

To facilitate healing, put pain management at the tippy-top of your priority list!

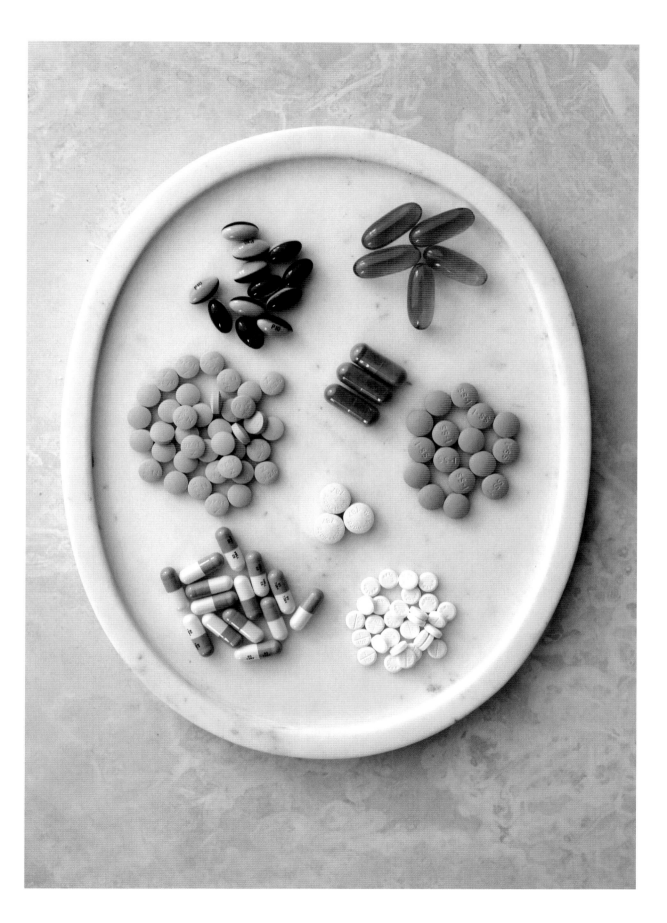

way—after a physical assault, your body immediately has two competing forces: pain and healing. Fundamentally, whichever jumps up and down and screams the loudest gets the attention. In most cases, this is pain (which means that healing gets cast off in order to deal with the pain).

However, when pain is managed or even alleviated, then your body can focus on healing. The bottom line is this: pain management promotes healing. So, which are you going to choose?

My final note about pain (though I could certainly go on and on and on!) deals with reasons that people avoid pain medication. I know so many people who have a fear of taking it. These fears are some of the biggest barriers to taking pain medicine or engaging in other pain-relieving modalities. "I'm so afraid of getting hooked," they say. Unless there is a prior history of addiction, this fear is completely and totally unfounded.

Back to the ceiling . . . it took a good fourteen-plus hours to get my pain under control enough that I could formulate cohesive sentences. Well, barely cohesive, anyway. This colossal screw-up that happened even with a nurse girlfriend in the room with me set me and my future treatment back at least a month, so much so, in fact, that breast cancer was almost completely out of my realm of thinking. In those subsequent weeks postsurgery, my life revolved around pain and other side effects (C.O.N.S.T.I.P.A.T.I.O.N.). Ultimately, my chemo was delayed for three weeks in order to get my pain and corresponding symptoms under some semblance of control.

Back to the hospital bed . . . after I came to my senses, I was able to begin to assess my postsurgical situation (though the bandages stayed on for several days). Four new appendages that I noticed immediately were the Jackson-Pratt drains, aka JP drains. A Jackson-Pratt drain is a surgical drainage device that removes excess fluid that can collect inside your body after surgery. When fluid builds up in a postsurgical site, the area may not heal as fast as it should or, even worse, the fluid can cause an infection. Too much fluid in a postsurgical area may also cause pain and swelling. Using a JP drain after surgery usually helps you heal faster and helps clear away pus. Yes, pus. I never said that this would be pretty.

A JP drain looks essentially like a plastic hand grenade. And I woke up with four of them. Yes, *four*. They were quite uncomfortable, not in a painful way but in an annoying, what-on-*earth*-is-sticking-out-of-me kind of way. When it came to sleeping, I felt like the princess from "The Princess and the Pea" . . . having to position myself just so. No matter what, though, I woke up in the middle of the night being jabbed by one of them. Good times.

JP drains are emptied (and contents measured) on average twice a day. The drains had to stay in place until less than 30 milliliters of fluid were drained from each in a day (cc's and milliliters are the same, by the way). In my case, this meant a week, which was not too bad at all, especially considering that some people have to keep them in for much longer.

During the first dressing change in the hospital (for which I was awake), I saw my new "breasts" (I called them "lady lumps") for the first time. They were a nice size (the same that I had before) and shape (perkier). They were also nipple-less and had incisions covered by Steri-Strips (small white strips of tape that hold the external stitches together). It was a shocker. Definitely. But, I figured that I had two choices about how to respond: I could be okay with my new "lady lumps" or I could not be okay. I chose okay.

The day after surgery, I knew I needed to get out of bed and move (even though I was still in a tremendous amount of pain). Though my body didn't want to move (because of the pain), Nurse LiFT said: "*Get up now*"—because the more you move, the more likely you are to prevent postoperative complications. The Silver Lining of moving is that it can help hasten your release from the hospital. So, I huffed and puffed my way down the hospital halls with my IV pole in tow.

Despite the abhorrent pain and constipation issues I had, I did remarkably well postsurgery and was scheduled to go home in three days, not four, which was a major Silver Lining. Prior to hospital discharge, the pathology results came back. More sobering news: my results demonstrated that my breast cancer was IIb, "multifocal, T1, N1," which translated to having multiple tumors in my right breast (we knew that already), each of which was 2 centimeters or less, and that my cancer had spread to my sentinel (underarm) lymph node. The spreading aspect was the suckiest part. The sentinel lymph node is the first node in a group of nodes where cancer cells may spread after they leave the original cancer site. The sentinel node for breast cancer is normally one of the lymph nodes under the arm. A sentinel lymph node biopsy (SLNB) is done to see if a known cancer has spread to lymph nodes.

> **LIFELINE**
>
> *The hospital sends you home with specific instructions on how to empty the drains. Most often a nurse can come to your home to do follow-up teaching (because heaven knows there is only so much a postsurgical brain can absorb!).*

> **LIFELINE**
>
> *Even though you may feel wretched & walking is the last thing you want to do after surgery, get up & M-O-V-E! The more you move, the faster you will heal.*

What this meant for me was that the breast cancer had spread out of the breast and into the lymph system. What this also meant for me was that the biggest and strongest of all chemotherapy regimens and radiation would be a definite part of my future.

That pathology result also showed that my type was ER/PR+, HER2-negative. ER/PR+ (estrogen and/or progesterone receptor positive) cancer means that the cancer cells grow in response to the presence of the hormones estrogen and/or progesterone. Approximately 75 percent of all types of breast cancer are ER+. HER2 (human epidermal growth factor receptor 2) is a gene that can be a factor in the development of breast cancer. In my case, because I was HER2-negative, HER2 did not play a role. Knowing my status helped my oncologist determine both the type of chemotherapy that I would need as well as the endocrine therapy that I would require after chemo.

A positive note on the pathology report was that the cancer was limited to my right breast. Even though I found out that there was no cancer in my left breast, I still felt like a double mastectomy was the right decision for me.

Upon hospital discharge, there was a *lot* to think about. To begin with, I was given a prescription for pain medication, as well as clear dosage instructions. My nurse suggested that I get this prescription filled as soon as possible to avoid uncontrolled pain during initial recovery. My sweet husband practically *ran* down to the outpatient pharmacy to get this prescription filled!

My nurse also told me that I was never, ever to have my blood pressure taken, an IV inserted into, or blood drawn from my right arm, the arm that had the axillary dissection (the surgical procedure that opened my armpit to identify, examine, and remove lymph nodes).

My surgeons instructed me to leave the bandages on my chest until I went to my initial follow-up visit. I was told that my surgical site was sutured with stitches that would dissolve (and would not need to be removed).

Additionally, I was told that because my mastectomy involved removal of lymph nodes in my armpit, I needed to be aware of the potential for lymphedema, which is characterized by swelling of the lymph tissue. My nurse also advised me to be aware of tightness in my arm, to refrain from wearing clingy clothes or jewelry on that arm, to avoid sun and insects, and to wait to exercise until I received clearance from my doctor (as if!).

I was also told to get extra rest and conserve my strength whenever possible. I am so glad that all of this information was written down, because I was way too fuzzy to get my head around much of anything, much less a long list of instructions!

Over the course of the next few weeks, my arms made nice progress in terms of mobility. My incisions healed very well and my JP drains were removed in a timely fashion, ten days after surgery. The big, ginormous bummer was my persistent pain. It took several weeks to get the pain under control; however, the Silver Lining was that I had the best, most creative palliative care team to lead the charge. ♥

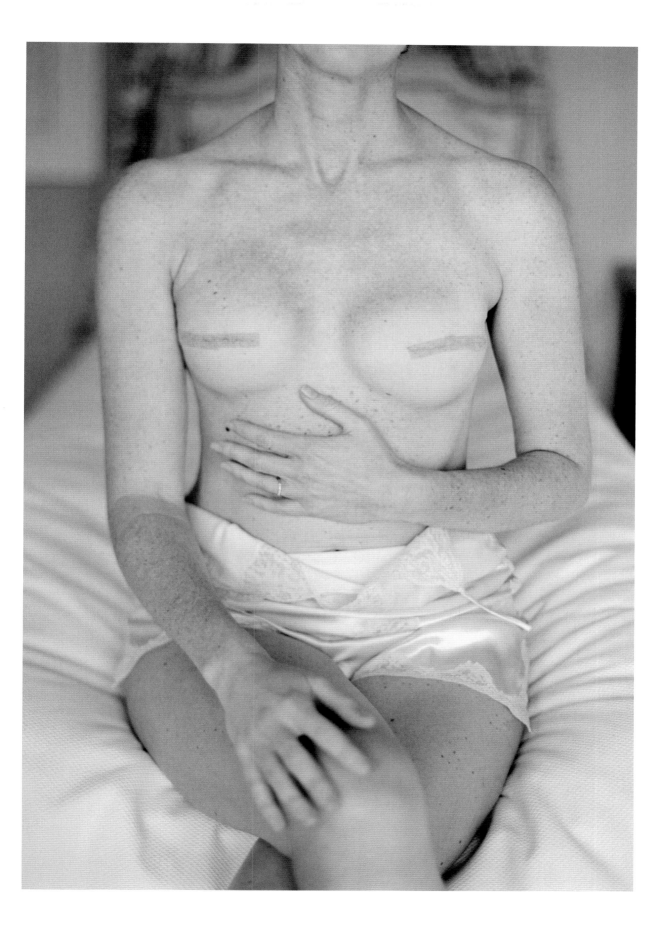

THE SILVER LINING

Between my diagnosis and surgery,

I felt overwhelmed, confused, and often lost.

It was as if I could not see the forest for the trees.

However, during recovery from surgery,

in spite of my exceptionally, extraordinarily,

unnecessarily long and difficult healing process,

I found some beautiful Silver Linings.

I learned that I am capable of things

I never could have imagined.

A disease diagnosis has the potential to bring out the

best in people (I have ignored the worst!).

Despite looking in the mirror and seeing mutilation

and illness, I knew in my heart that

I was still Me.

No surgery or disease could take that away from me.

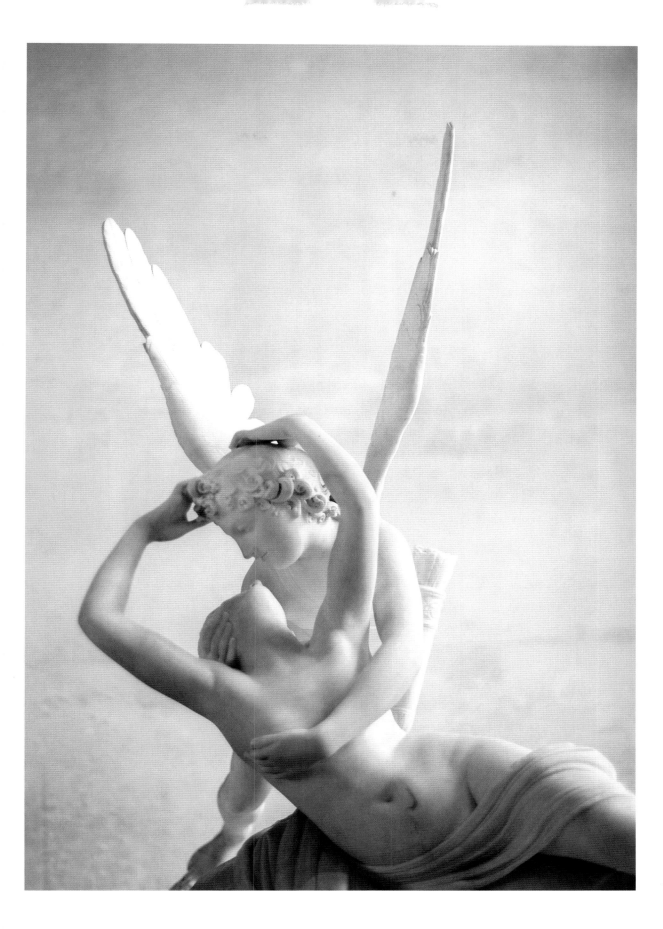

Support & Suggestions

- When it comes to making decisions, make them when they need to be made. I made the mistake of thinking that I had to make all decisions about treatment (Surgery? Chemotherapy? Radiation?) at the time of my diagnosis. Not even close. My first priorities needed to be hiring my surgeons, figuring out additional tests I needed, and making a plan for surgery. Decisions about chemotherapy and radiation could wait.

- The shock of seeing my new "lady lumps" after surgery wasn't nearly as bad as I thought it was going to be.

- One of the postsurgical side effects of a double mastectomy and reconstruction is arm immobility. In other words, it took a tremendous amount of painful stretching to get motion back into my arms, because for five weeks my arms were predominantly at my side (as instructed by my impressively conservative plastic surgeon). There are some physical therapists who are trained to help with mobility after a mastectomy. Be sure to consult with your surgeon(s) prior to working with anyone, though!

- Before and after surgery, I increased my protein intake to promote healing and to promote wound healing.

- The second you see someone coming in to give you a hug, put your hands up and *stop* them. It took me almost six months before I could give/get a pain-free hug!

- Plan for food when you get home. Though you won't feel like eating, it will be a necessity when taking pain medicine. This is a great way to engage family and friends who want to help.

- If you don't have someone staying with you in the hospital, arrange for a ride home and ideally a person to help get you settled at home.

- Ask your breast surgeon(s) if nursing services are available for home health. I had a nurse come several times a week after my surgery to check on my wounds and drains and to help me shower.

People You May See in Your Planning Process

- breast surgeons
- doctors who specialize in diagnostic tests, such as mammograms (radiologists)
- doctors who specialize in treating cancer (oncologists)
- doctors who treat cancer with radiation (radiation oncologists)
- genetic counselors
- plastic surgeons
- fertility specialists (if you are contemplating having a baby after treatment)

Questions to Ask Your Doctors

Diagnosis/Testing

Some of the questions below are also in the first chapter, but I found that asking the same questions multiple times helped me find clarity.

1. What exactly is my diagnosis?
2. What are the stage and grade (aggressiveness) of my cancer?
3. What can you tell me about my tumor(s) (e.g., the size, estrogen receptor status)?
4. Would you explain my test results to me? May I have a copy for my records? (Sometimes institutions charge to have copies made.)
5. Do I need any more tests? If so, what, why, and when?
6. Has the cancer metastasized (spread) to any other site? If so, where?
7. What are the results of my sentinel node biopsy?

Treatment

1. What treatment options are available for me?
2. What are your specific recommendations?
3. How do you decide which treatments to recommend?
4. What is the evidence for your recommendations?
5. What are the benefits from each treatment you recommend?
6. What are the likely and/or possible side effects of each treatment option?
7. What are the possible risks, both short-term and long-term?
8. Will treatment impact my ability to have a child after treatment? If so, how? Would you refer me to a fertility specialist?
9. Where will treatments be given? How often? What is the duration?
10. How will each treatment affect my daily life? Can I continue working?
11. How quickly do I need to make a decision about cancer treatment?
12. What happens if I don't want cancer treatment?
13. What will cancer treatment cost?
14. Does my insurance plan cover the tests and treatment you're recommending?
15. I will be getting a second opinion. Is it better to get a second opinion now before any treatments begin, or wait until after all of the tests are complete?
16. What can I do to manage or avoid lymphedema?
17. Are there any brochures or other printed material that I can take with me?
18. What websites or books would you recommend to learn more?
19. Is cancer rehabilitation an option from the time I begin treatment?

What to Take to Appointments

- journal and/or computer for taking notes
- a person to support you and help take notes
- your list of questions
- insurance information
- your comprehensive medical-record copy and any pathology reports
- films or digital images of any previous PET exams, X-rays, CTs, or MRI scans

Mastectomy Types*

SIMPLE (TOTAL) MASTECTOMY: Surgical removal of one or both breasts, including the areola and nipple, as well as some of the overlying skin; however, the adjacent lymph nodes and chest muscles are left intact.

MODIFIED RADICAL MASTECTOMY: The surgical removal of the entire breast or breasts, including the skin, breast tissue, areola, and nipple. Most of the lymph nodes under the arm

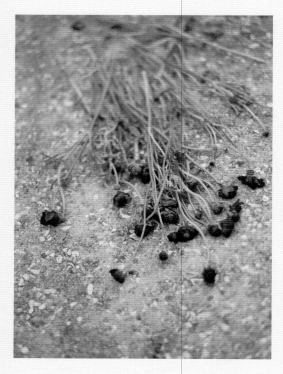

are also removed; however, the pectoralis major muscle is spared. This is what I had. The procedure may be followed by reconstruction (as was the case with me).

RADICAL MASTECTOMY: The surgical removal of one or both breasts, underlying pectoralis major and pectoralis minor chest muscles, and many of the lymph nodes under the arm (the axilla). This is no longer a commonly performed procedure.

PROPHYLACTIC MASTECTOMY: The surgical removal of one or both breasts before disease develops, in hopes of avoiding future disease.

SEGMENTAL MASTECTOMY (PARTIAL MASTECTOMY/LUMPECTOMY): A breast-conserving surgery that removes the part of the breast with the cancer and some of the surrounding normal tissue.

Adapted from breastcancer.org, used with permission.

SUBCUTANEOUS (NIPPLE-SPARING) MASTECTOMY: Surgical removal of only the underlying breast tissue. The breast skin, areola, and nipple remain. Must be accompanied by immediate breast reconstruction. This type of mastectomy is done less frequently because the tissue that is left behind could develop cancer at a later time.

Reconstruction Types*

AUTOLOGOUS RECONSTRUCTION uses tissue—skin, fat, and sometimes muscle—from another place on your body to form a breast shape. Examples include:

- TRAM flap: Short for "transverse rectus abdominis myocutaneous." Uses tissue from the patient's lower abdomen to reconstruct the surgically removed breast. The lower abdomen tissue remains attached to the central abdominal muscles, maintaining blood flow to the transferred tissue.

- DIEP flap: Short for "deep inferior epigastric perforator." Uses the tissue from the patient's lower abdomen to reconstruct the surgically removed breast; however, unlike the TRAM procedure, no muscle is sacrificed.

- SIEA flap: Named for the superficial inferior epigastric artery blood vessel that runs just under your skin in your lower abdomen. It is similar to a DIEP flap; however, a different section of blood vessels in the belly are moved with the fat and skin. Additionally, the SIEA flap does not require that a small incision be made in the rectus abdominis muscle.

- Latissimus dorsi flap: Uses muscle and skin tunneled from the back of the shoulder blade to reconstruct the surgically removed breast. Additional surgery is required to create a nipple and areola.

- GAP flap: Uses the gluteal artery perforator blood vessel that runs through the buttocks as well as a section of skin and fat from the buttocks to reconstruct the breast.

IMPLANT RECONSTRUCTION uses an implant to rebuild the breast. This was the best option for me because I am thin and had small breasts. Implants can be filled with saline (salt water), silicone gel, or a combination of the two, with silicone in the outside chamber and saline on the inside. What I liked about this type of surgery was that the length of surgery and recovery time were shorter.

* Adapted from breastcancer.org, used with permission.

Some Presurgical Tests

EKG: To give a preliminary indication of how well your heart is functioning.

BLOOD TEST: To assess for any infection and how well your organs are functioning.

URINALYSIS: To determine how well your kidneys are functioning.

PHYSICAL THERAPY EVALUATION: To assess your arm mobility before surgery and then have a frame of reference for after surgery. Though I didn't do it, I wish that I had, because I ended up seeing a physical therapist after surgery who asked all kinds of questions (that I couldn't answer) about my mobility before surgery. The Silver Lining is that you can learn from me!

Surgery Packing List

COMFY BUTTON-FRONT PAJAMAS One size larger than you usually wear and the softer the better.

DRY SHAMPOO Because I knew that I wasn't going to be able to shower.

BRUSH Ask a friend to brush your hair after surgery because it feels so doggone good!

LIP BALM AND MOISTURIZER Because patients in the hospital are forever feeling parched.

BABY WIPES A great thing to have to help with cleanliness, especially when you don't want to get up to go to the bathroom.

GLASSES It's so much easier to forgo contacts while in the hospital.

MINTS Because anesthesia makes your breath pretty amazingly stinky, even after you've brushed your teeth.

TRAVEL TOOTHBRUSH With a cap on it to avoid the omnipresent germs of a hospital.

A SOFT BLANKET So much better than any blanket covering in the hospital.

ENTERTAINMENT Movies on your tablet, books and magazines, the more entertaining the better.

CAMISOLE WITH JP DRAIN POUCH Not remotely attractive, but the Silver Lining is that it's functional!

POSTSURGERY BREAST TRAVEL PILLOW Absolutely necessary for any and every car ride; place it between you and the upper-body part of the seat belt to distribute pressure on your chest—mine had a Velcro loop on one side of the pillow so that I could attach it to the seat belt.

GOING-HOME OUTFIT Leggings and an extra-large men's shirt that buttons in the front—I took a cast-off from my husband's closet; these clothes will get schmutz—blood, postsurgical fluid—on them; this is not the time for fancy!

SOFT SOCKS AND SLIPPERS To keep your feet warm and for walking the halls of the hospital.

Preoperative Instructions

I was told:

- Do not take aspirin or aspirin-containing products for ten days before surgery. Tylenol is okay. Stop taking vitamin E supplements two weeks before your surgery or as soon as possible.
- You will need blood work, a urinalysis, and an EKG the week before surgery (to ensure that your body's organs can handle the rigors of surgery).
- Do not eat or drink anything after midnight on the night before your surgery.
- Plan to be in the hospital for anywhere between two and four days.
- You will need to have a responsible adult to drive you home . . . and don't plan on driving for at least a month.

Postoperative Instructions

I was told to call my doctor if I had any of the following:

- pain that is not relieved by medication
- fever more than 100 degrees Fahrenheit or chills
- excessive bleeding, such as a bloody dressing
- excessive swelling
- redness outside the dressing
- discharge or bad odor from the wound
- allergic or other reactions to medication(s)
- constipation
- anxiety, depression, trouble sleeping, or needed more support. *Ha!* As if anxiety, depression, trouble sleeping, and the need for more support were unusual after you've had your breasts amputated!
- Additionally, I was instructed to empty the fluid from the JP drain at least twice a day and record the amount of fluid collected every day.

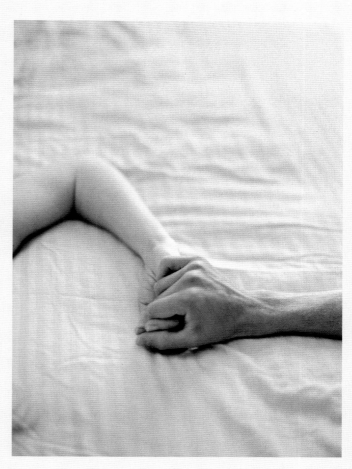

CHAPTER IV
Chemo Sobby
The Experience of Chemotherapy

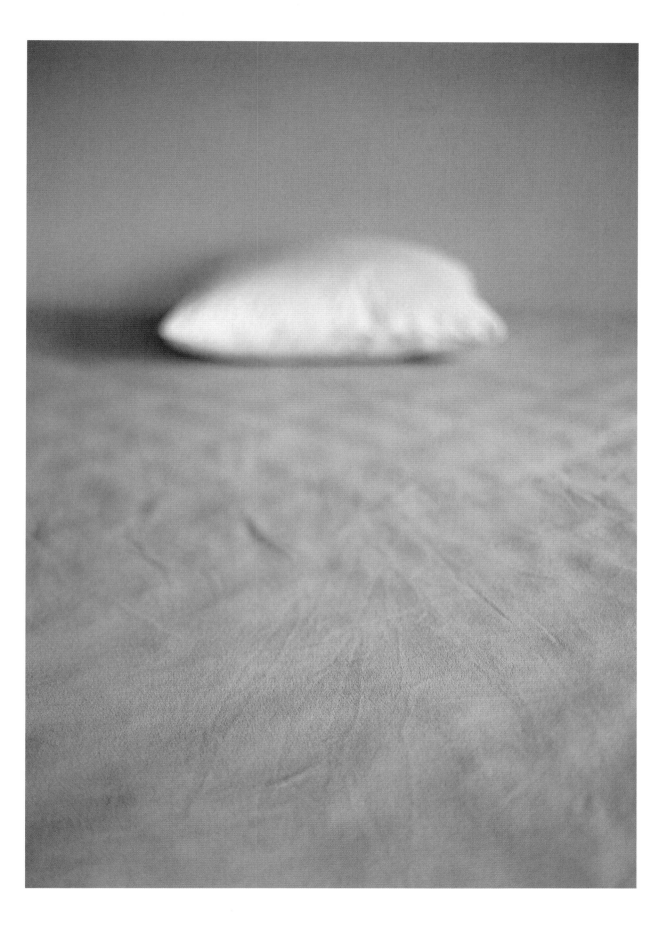

here's something about breast cancer that induces naive delusions. I figured that after my out-of-left-field diagnosis and ridiculous surgical experience, I would get a break, that chemotherapy would be tolerable. "Ha! Ha! Ha!" said breast cancer.

DECISION FATIGUE

One of the many challenges of navigating the world of health care after a cancer diagnosis is that there are a trillion decisions to make (at least it feels this way!). These options are seemingly informed by millions of people with gazillions of opinions. This, combined with the fact that medicine is often equal parts science and art, I (even as a nurse!) found myself overwhelmed and exhausted emotionally, mentally, and physically. There were days when even the teeniest decision sent me into a full meltdown. White shirt? Blue shirt? *Argh!*

Research has shown that "decision fatigue" is physiologically real. In other words, it wasn't in my imagination. Social psychologists describe decision fatigue as difficulty in making good decisions late in the day, or when people have had to make a series of choices in a short period of time, as is the case after a breast cancer diagnosis. Decision fatigue means that brain energy for choices is depleted and any important decision we make runs the risk of being flawed. This information was a major Silver Lining for me because I often thought that I was losing my mind when I couldn't make the smallest decision.

Decision fatigue is not limited to illness. When you think about it, most people routinely make gobs of decisions every day. Each and every decision takes a dollop of brain power. Add in a stressful doctor's appointment, for example, and the ability to think clearly and weigh options wisely declines.

In a *New York Times* article, John Tierney explored the causes and impact of decision fatigue. The article reviewed recent data that confirm that the complexity of making choices or decisions can be very fatiguing. In fact, he suggests that the very act of making a decision exacts a "biological cost." When I read this, I began nodding my head (and didn't stop until the end of the article):

> No matter how rational and high-minded you try to be, you can't make decision after decision without paying a biological price. It's different from ordinary physical fatigue—you're not consciously aware of being tired—but you're low on mental energy. The more choices you make throughout the day, the harder each one becomes for your brain, and eventually it looks for shortcuts, usually in either of two very different ways. One shortcut is to become reckless: to act impulsively instead

of expending the energy to first think through the consequences. The other shortcut is the ultimate energy saver: do nothing. Instead of agonizing over decisions, avoid any choice.

So, as we make decisions throughout the day, our brains become fatigued, and either we act impulsively and choose unwisely or even take unnecessary risks, or we avoid making any decision at all. Consequently, this has a direct effect on our ability to continue to make *good* decisions.

What's also interesting is that researchers discovered (by accident!) that when our brains have been making lots of choices, we also run low on glucose. The Silver Lining is that, according to recent research findings, a shot of glucose helps the brain overcome decision-fatigue and restore some ability to think clearly (no, this doesn't mean a face plant in a bag of chocolate—sorry!).

The implications for people diagnosed with breast cancer or other potentially life-threatening illness are clear. Serious illness involves myriad choices to be made, often in quick succession. The decision fatigue research shows that it is not necessarily the magnitude of decisions but the quantity of them that causes fatigue. As if it's not already difficult enough, further adding to decision fatigue, patients and families have to figure out how to navigate the complex health care system, from where to park at the health care facility to how to deal with insurance issues. This is why it's important to build a team: to help you make decisions.

COUTURE CHEMO

While certain types of cancers have predictable treatments, many factors go into creating an individual's specific, customized treatment plan. The majority of the considerations come from the pathophysiology of the disease—in other words, studying the mechanical, physiological, and biochemical aspects of each diagnosis. Pathology reports are usually created both at the time of the original biopsy and at the time of surgery (to ensure a corroborative diagnosis). Results can take several days. Why? Well, since cancer is a genetic mutation that results in an abnormal growth of cells, the process involves multiple tests, analysis, and consultation among specialists.

A few weeks after my surgery, my husband and I met with our newly hired, pro–palliative care oncologist. In preparing for our first meeting, we—yes, you guessed it—came up with a list of questions the night before our appointment. Notice I said "we" . . . as a reminder that it is always best to go to an appointment with someone.

Preparing questions gives you the framework

LIFELINE

The period of waiting for test results can be excruciating. Distract yourself in peaceful ways: take a walk, meditate, or listen to music.

for structured, organized discussion and ensures that all of your questions are answered. When we walked into the oncologist's office for our meeting, the first thing that I noticed was a sign above his desk that read, EVERY JOURNEY BRINGS BLESSINGS. I thought, "This is definitely the right guy for the job."

Equipped with our list of questions, knowing that I was stage IIb, I braced myself for the harsh reality that I was actually discussing chemotherapy . . . going Into-My-Body. It was surreal. My compensatory mechanism at every doctor's appointment happened to be a functional one; I pulled out my list of questions and laptop to take notes.

1. **DO I REALLY NEED CHEMOTHERAPY?** Duh.

2. **WILL I TAKE AN ONCOTYPE DX TEST?** No, because my cancer had invaded the lymph system. Depending on a patient's staging (if stage I or II invasive breast cancer), hormone receptor status (if estrogen positive), lymph node involvement (if none), your oncologist may order an Oncotype DX test before treatment begins. This test provides valuable information about whether you need chemo by assessing how likely a tumor is to grow, the likelihood that the tumor would respond to treatment, and the likelihood of recurrence. Once my breast cancer spread to my lymph nodes, chemotherapy was a guaranteed sure thing.

3. **WHAT TYPE OF CHEMOTHERAPY?** TAC, which encompasses:

   a. docetaxel, which is known by the trade name Taxotere—this drug prevents cancer cells from dividing and therefore reproducing;

   b. doxorubicin is known by the trade name Adriamycin—this drug gets inside the DNA of cancer cells and prevents cell replication by inhibiting protein synthesis;

   c. cyclophosphamide, also known by the trade name Cytoxan—this drug breaks the DNA of cancer cells so they can't keep dividing, and they die.

4. **HOW MANY DRUGS?** Three chemotherapy drugs (as described above) plus a shot of Neulasta twenty-four hours after each dose of chemotherapy. Pegfilgrastim, which is known by the trade name Neulasta is given to reduce the risk of infection in patients receiving chemotherapy.

5. **WHY THE DIFFERENT DRUGS?** The reason for multiple drugs is because of the wacky but highly sophisticated cellular makeup of a tumor. One tumor can have many different types of cells in it. Some of these cells may have extra chromosomes, different growth rates, and varying sensitivity to chemotherapeutic agents. Therefore, the goal is to give enough different medications to affect all of the different types of cells in the tumor(s).

6. HOW MANY CYCLES? Six cycles.

7. WHAT IS THE TIMING FOR MEDICATION DELIVERY? Every three weeks for four months.

8. WILL I GET RADIATION? At the time, there was a very strong likelihood that I would *not* have to have radiation; however, if you've read the table of contents, you'll know how that turned out for me.

9. HOW CAN I INCORPORATE COMPLEMENTARY MEDICINE? Lots of ways, including acupuncture, reflexology, moxibustion, nutrition, meditation, music therapy, reiki, aromatherapy, physical therapy, and yoga.

10. WILL I GET A PORT-A-CATH? Yes, because I wanted one. A PORT-A-CATH is a small medical device that facilitates the administration of chemotherapy into the veins. It is a fabulous gadget that is used to make the administration of chemotherapy and blood draws easier because it is designed to permit repeated access to the venous system. It can also reduce the risk of certain chemotherapy side effects. A PORT-A-CATH is placed under the skin, typically in the upper part of the chest. Having cared for people with PORT-A-CATHs and people without, I knew without a doubt that I wanted one! A Silver Lining of a PORT-A-CATH is that people can resume regular activities, including swimming and other exercise and sports; however, I was advised to avoid contact sports. Too bad.

> **LIFELINE**
>
> *Not everyone chooses to have a PORT-A-CATH. It really is up to you. What I know for sure is that I'm really happy that I did!*

PRE-CHEMO TO-DO LIST

The first thing that I did after that appointment was to schedule my PORT-A-CATH insertion (which is a minor surgical procedure). My oncologist planned on having several days between its placement and my first chemo infusion, though it is possible to have chemo on the same day that a PORT-A-CATH is placed. As we left this appointment, I felt as if I had nerve bugs in my tummy. I wasn't scared (though not because I was extraordinarily brave), but nervous. Nervous about how my physical body was going to react to the medications.

In addition to scheduling my PORT-A-CATH placement, I made an appointment with my palliative care team. Why did I need to see them (some people continued to ask)? Well, because they were an invaluable part of my team who had a great role in getting my postsurgical pain and constipation under contol. *Hellooo?* Who *wouldn't* have palliative care as part of her health care team?

During this palliative care appointment, I had two ongoing issues with which I needed postsurgical assistance. The first issue was the heightened, alarmlike state that my lady lumps were constantly in. This is explained clinically as neuropathy. When nerves are damaged (as mine unavoidably were during the surgery), the changes in the remaining part of the nerve result in heightened sensitivity. (This was a bit

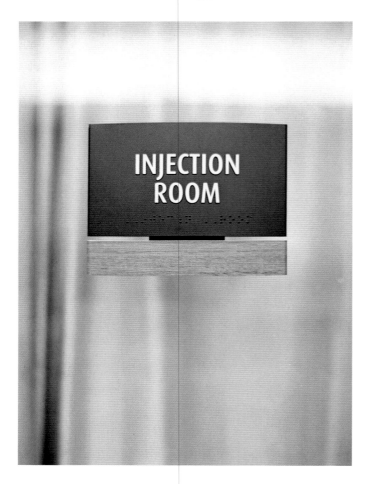

of an understatement. They felt as if they were on edge, incredibly raw, and outrageously tender. To pass a Q-tip across them was excruciating!) My doctor gave me a good analogy; it was like having repeated seizures in my lady lumps. Therefore, he prescribed a drug called Neurontin (the generic name is "gabapentin") to offset these totally unacceptable seizurelike activities. A Silver Lining of this drug is that it can also be used to treat and prevent hot flashes in women who are being treated for breast cancer. Oh yes, a little teaser of what was to come.

The second issue we discussed was my wellness program. Yes, for all those naysayers, palliative care *does* do wellness programs! This included the things that I could actively do to keep my head and heart as together as possible throughout the process: guided meditation, restorative yoga, and music therapy, to name a few.

Next on the pre-chemo to-do list was an appointment for an echocardiogram. An echocardiogram (sometimes called an ECHO) is a heart test procedure that uses a probe (called a transducer) to send high-frequency sound waves into your chest. These sound waves bounce (or echo) off your heart. A computer uses the "echo" sound waves to create a moving picture of your heart to analyze how well it functions. ECHOs are prescribed because some chemotherapy drugs can cause temporary damage to the muscles of the heart, which may change the rhythm of the heartbeat. If this happens, most people go back to normal after the treatment has ended. This procedure is painless. I found a Silver Lining in that my heart was functioning normally.

As I was preparing myself physically and cognitively, I felt more and more anxiety. So much of it had to do with not knowing how my body would respond. I eased my nerve bugs by looking for Silver Linings. These did not in any way, shape, or form negate the harsh reality of what I was facing, but they did provide perspective and balance. One Silver Lining came when I talked with friends who had gone through chemo. Though there were a couple of exceptions, most people I asked said that they "breezed" through chemo with few side effects and the ability to maintain a fairly normal life. By normal, I mean that they were able to work, maintain their households, and even spend time with friends. They just did these things bald and a little more tired. I aspired to have the same response.

Another Silver Lining was that I knew I had an incredible, professional team of caregivers who made me feel safe and secure. I knew that if the side effects came and if they were as rotten as they could be, I would not have to manage them on my own. Though the anxiety was still there, the Silver Lined perspective of knowing that I was not alone gave me strength and courage.

My personal and professional philosophy has always been: Hope for the best. Prepare for the worst.

THE FIRST CHEMO

The night before my first dose of chemo, I packed a bag to take with me. You would have thought that I was going on vacation for a few days because I brought a sweater and blanket (because hospitals and treatment areas are always cold!). For entertainment, I brought magazines, my iPad, my laptop, and a book. For nourishment, I brought healthy snacks (almonds, banana, and bottled water), and I brought my journal. Seriously, where on earth did I think I was going? Well, I'm glad I packed all that, because I used *everything* in my bag!

The morning of my first chemo, I woke up with my anxiety on high alert. My husband, who by this time I had renamed the HOTY (Husband of the Year), came with me to chemo. Boy oh boy did he ever earn his title. Not only did he come to chemo but he came to literally every single solitary appointment with me, from surgery to blood draws. He was, and continues to be, the greatest Silver Lining *ever*.

I was the first patient that morning at the Cancer Center of Santa Barbara. At the reception desk, I was given a pink questionnaire that asked about any symptoms I was currently experiencing. "Huh?" I wondered. I hadn't even started yet. When I inquired about why I had to fill out the form, considering I hadn't had my first drop of chemo, I was told that it was standard protocol before every chemotherapy infusion. After a five-minute wait (which felt like an eternity), I was escorted to the treatment room. It was a beautiful, spacious, and calm place.

Three nurses introduced themselves. All were very welcoming and kind. I even had my pick of chairs. Woo-hoo! We discussed accessing my PORT-A-CATH. "Accessing" a PORT-A-CATH means putting a large Huber needle into it. Connected to the needle is an IV line through which chemotherapy and other medications are administered.

I told the nurses that thanks to my abhorrent postmastectomy pain management, I had an extremely *low* tolerance for pain, that even the lightest touch hurt. I requested both Lidocaine and EMLA cream. EMLA cream is a local anesthetic (comprised of lidocane 2.5% and prilocaine 2.5%) that numbs the skin before needle insertion. It works by blocking nerves from transmitting painful impulses to the brain. They didn't have any at the treatment center. To get EMLA cream, you need a doctor's prescription and it takes an hour to take effect. *Ugh.* At this point, I really wasn't sure how much more I could take.

Okay, well, how about a little injectable Lidocaine to numb the area? I asked.

Nope. They didn't have that either. Really? I almost broke into tears. I reiterated exactly how low my tolerance for pain was and they promised to do it as fast as possible.

All I can say is that accessing my PORT-A-CATH was a disaster and felt like: *Alarm! Alarm! Alarm! Owie! Owie! Owie!* Holy heavens. Tears instantly poured down my cheeks. I wanted to throw up. It was *awful*. Not only that, but the nurse didn't hit the bull's-eye and had to pull it out and do it *again*.

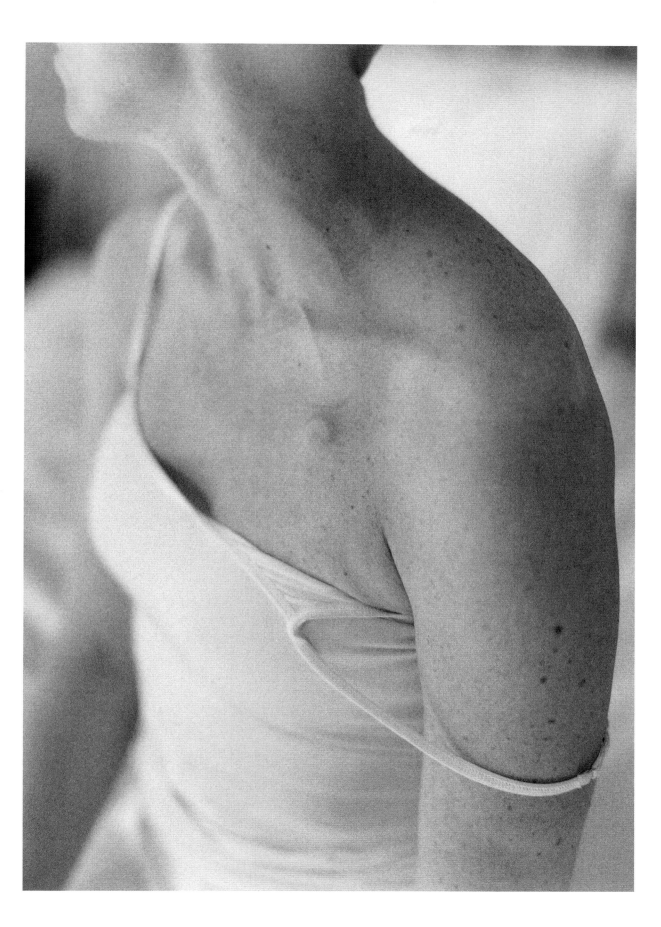

The poor nurse was mortified and completely apologetic, while I was nearly apoplectic. It was awful all the way around. She *finally* hit the center of the port and was able to get fluids to go through. Yeah!

Before chemo can be administered, blood must be drawn back through a syringe connected to the IV line. This ensures that the line is in the right place. Well, that didn't work initially either. So, she gave me two small bags of normal saline (salt water) to see whether fluids running through the IV for a short period of time could get the holy grail of blood to pull back in the syringe. Well, *finally* it worked. Yipppeee! Now we were ready to roll!

In the meantime, she also gave me intravenous Benadryl (to offset side effects, with the added bonus of making me sleepy) as well as Ativan (an antianxiety medication).

LIFELINE

Some people are supersensitive to the saline smell & can actually taste it. I recommend sucking on a mint or spraying lavender into a cloth & holding it to your nose as the line is being flushed with saline.

After I was given these two drugs, the steroid dexamethasone was administered through my IV. "Dex," as it's commonly called, helps prevent or minimize nausea and vomiting and increase appetite. On the opposite end of the spectrum, it can produce sleepless nights and anger issues, commonly referred to as 'roid rage. Ohhhhh, did I ever learn about 'roid rage.

Then, my doctor came into the room to tell me that there had been a "snafu."

LIFELINE

Prepare yourself & your loved ones for 'roid rage. I felt like a drunk & angry bull in a china shop. It was not pretty!

"What on *earth* is going on today? You've *got* to be kidding me," I thought. 'Roid rage was clearly beginning to take effect. The day before chemo, I was supposed to have taken dexamethasone by mouth. Really? *Really?* Hmmm . . . why didn't I, the patient, know this? So, because I did not have a dose of dex the day before treatment, I was unable to have my first dose of chemotherapy. My situation was a classic example of a patient falling through the cracks.

I would have to go back to the Cancer Center the following morning to try it again. Get back on the horse, as they say (but this time I'd have EMLA and antiemetics—anti-vomiting drugs—in my saddle)! I had to look *long and hard* for Silver Linings that day (especially considering the ever-mounting 'roid rage), but was able to find several:

1. I was able to get out all of the initial worries and anxieties about going to a cancer center to receive chemotherapy.
2. I got a prescription for EMLA cream to place on my PORT-A-CATH before the next day's stick.

3. I now knew what to expect when I went in for chemo.

4. My oncologist apologized profusely and could not have been more compassionate or supportive.

The next morning, after my trial run, I woke up feeling so much more calm and confident. Before I left for the clinic, I took three medications:

1. **ATIVAN** to relieve anxiety. Ativan slows activity in the brain to allow for relaxation. Though I already felt like my brain activity was slow, it did indeed do the relaxation trick.

2. **EMEND** to prevent nausea and vomiting caused by chemotherapy. Be sure to take this *before* chemo because it doesn't stop nausea and vomiting after they start.

3. **EMLA CREAM** on my PORT-A-CATH to prevent the pain associated with the needle stick.

> ### LIFELINE
> *Put a generous amount of EMLA cream on one hour before the PORT-A-CATH is accessed. Don't be bashful about it. I frequently glopped it on & then covered it gently with a tissue so that the cream didn't get on my clothes.*

When I got to the clinic, they were all *fully* prepared. Phew. What a relief. The first step was inserting the Huber needle into my EMLA-laden PORT-A-CATH. The Silver Lining of my day was that my nurse accessed my PORT-A-CATH on the first try. There really is no way to describe the joy that brought me.

Before administering chemotherapy, I had to have the following three pre-chemo IV medications:

1. **ALOXI** to prevent nausea and vomiting that may occur within twenty-four hours after receiving cancer chemotherapy. It is also used to prevent delayed nausea and vomiting that may occur several days after receiving certain chemotherapy medications.

2. **DECADRON** (aka dex): to relieve inflammation in various parts of the body, treat or prevent allergic reactions, treat nausea and vomiting associated with some chemotherapy drugs, and stimulate appetite in cancer patients with severe appetite problems. So, not only did I have to take it by mouth the night before chemo, but I had to have another dose by IV just before chemo.

3. **BENADRYL** to prevent and reverse nausea. It can also cause mild relaxation, drowsiness, dry mouth, and constipation.

> ### LIFELINE
> *If you take Benadryl, be prepared to take Senokot & MiraLAX. Stay AHEAD of constipation!!!!*

After all of the above drugs were given, it was time for my first dose of chemotherapy. The drugs are often given one at a time, in order to assess potential allergic reactions.

1. **TAXOTERE** was the first drug because it is the most likely to produce immediate side effects (such as shortness of breath). Fortunately I had none, which was a Silver Lining!
2. **ADRIAMYCIN** (aka "the Red Devil"—seriously, I could not have possibly made that up!) came next. This drug has to be hand-pushed slowly into the PORT-A-CATH because if the medication leaks out of the tubing, it can be seen immediately. Another Silver Lining, no leakages!
3. **CYTOXAN** was the third drug. It is administered over the course of thirty minutes. I was told, "Let anyone know if you get any congestion issues"—which, thankfully, I didn't.

After three and a half hours of chemo preparation and then infusion, I was *done* with round one! I felt very sleepy from the Benadryl and the Ativan, but also incredibly grateful that everything went so smoothly!

Upon my returning home, Lalee found the Band-Aid covering my port totally unacceptable. She promptly changed my bandage to a Cinderella Band-Aid. She put it on so carefully and gently, but not before telling me to "be brave." As a result, she felt important and involved, which was an added Silver Lining of my day.

SIDE EFFECTS

When it came to side effects, I managed to have virtually *every* side effect of *every* drug. Now there is a really, really big Silver Lining to the fact that I was the Side Effects Queen: I am now able to share these effects with you from both a personal and professional perspective. In other words, I hope that you can learn from what I did well . . . and from what I didn't do so well.

The morning after my first round of chemo, I felt horrendous . . . as if I had been run over by a train and then thrown off a cliff. Thanks to the side effects of Decadron, when I looked in the mirror, my face was so red and flushed that it appeared as if I'd spent the day on the beach in Boca (in July!) sans sunscreen. *Ewwwwww!!*

Despite taking all of the prescribed anti-nausea drugs, I still wanted to heave every minute of every hour of every day. My mind was going in circles without formu-

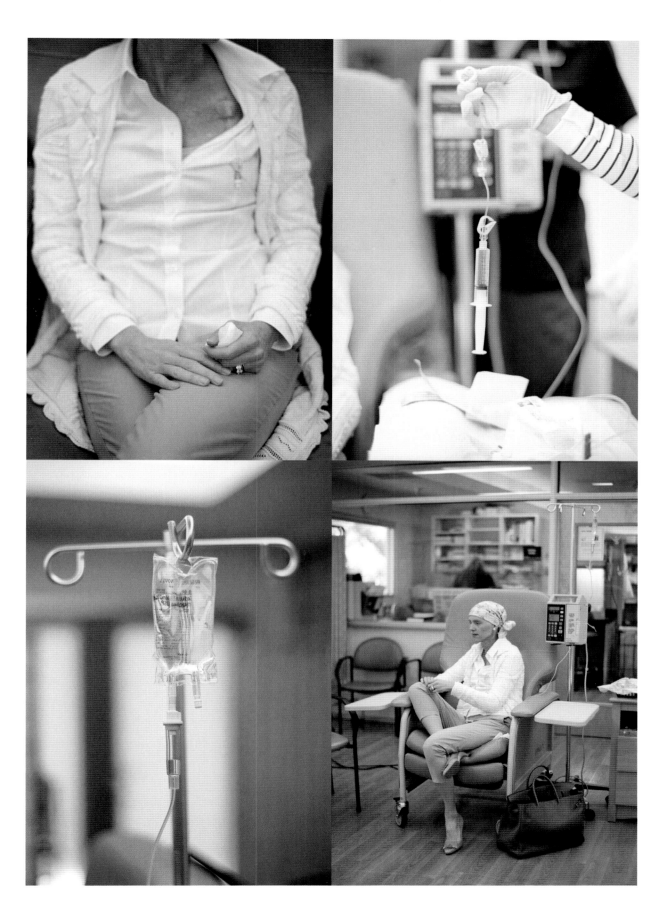

lating a single cohesive thought. *And* . . . the thought of moving my big toe to start the process of standing up was, well, exhausting.

Twenty-four hours after every chemo infusion, I went back to the clinic for a shot of a drug called Neulasta. One gnarly side effect of chemotherapy is that it has the potential to decrease the number of neutrophils (a type of blood cell needed to fight infection). Neulasta is a Silver Lining medication used to reduce the chance of infection. Neulasta comes as a solution (liquid) to inject subcutaneously (under the skin).

LIFELINE

Be very careful to avoid infection during chemo; wash your hands all day long!

With yet another drug comes yet another batch of (potential, though in my case realized) side effects, including bone pain, muscle pain, headaches, joint pain, vomiting, weakness, swelling or water retention in ankles or feet, and constipation. Really? *Again* with the constipation? I felt like some terrible digestive joke was being played on me.

Insurance covered the cost of this drug as it did for most of my medication. Thankfully. Speaking of insurance, not a day goes by that I don't think about the people in this country who either are underinsured or have no insurance at all. As if dealing with breast cancer (or any kind of cancer) isn't difficult enough. Anyhoo, after all of my clinical work, I found myself feeling especially grateful for my insurance. For those under- or un-insured, there is help!

Despite feeling putrid, I found a few more Silver Linings that day because I just couldn't help myself.

1. Being sick during the winter in California enabled me to go outside and warm my achy muscles and bones.
2. A dear friend dropped off homemade matzo ball soup without being asked. Turns out that it was the only thing I could eat that day!
3. I had a good, cleansing cry with a friend who didn't try to fix anything. She was just there for me.

INSOMNIA

During the course of my chemo treatment, I had many middle-of-the-night musings. Thanks to taking Decadron, I found myself up in the middle of the night without any hope of going back to sleep. Here's how it usually went: at some point in the middle of the night, my beloved dog, Buzz, and I headed out to watch the Tennis Channel. I love watching tennis almost as much as I love playing it. Old tournaments. Current tournaments. Grand Slams. Weird multicolored doubles competitions. It doesn't matter as long as a ball keeps going back and forth across the net.

To my utter chagrin, many nights I turned on the Tennis Channel only to find infomercials. Case in point: Ninja Kitchen System blender. The what? Yes, the Ninja Kitchen System blender. It makes peanut butter cookies *and* vegetable juice—at the same time. Uh-huh, that's what they told me. I think. All I wanted to do was watch some tennis. But *no,* I felt that my nutty-spinning-mushy-feeling brain was even more cuckoo than it was when I got up. The Silver Lining was that I did *not* buy anything during these middle-of-the-night marathon infomercial sessions (only because I couldn't find my credit card!).

Why didn't I read a book? you ask. Well, that would imply putting words together—in a row—to make sense of a story. Weekly gossip magazines might as well have been Dostoyevsky. It went like this night after night.

I found Silver Linings when I went outside and looked at the stars or listened to the soothing rain. Another Silver Lining was that though the hours were long, the nights went fast. Please don't ask me to explain that because I wouldn't have the slightest clue where to begin.

THE COMMODES I HAVE KNOWN

Five days after my first round of chemo, the HOTY and I went to LA for an appointment with my plastic surgeon and to proactively shop for a wig. A little sleepover getaway sounds nice, right?

Could it possibly have been that easy-breezy? *Naaaaaaaah.* Not a chance.

As you all may remember (or willfully have forgotten), after my surgery, I had some major (*major*) plumbing problems . . . as in nonfunction. Total shutdown. Zippo action. After chemo, I found myself with the opposite problem. O.P.P.O.S.I.T.E. I know it's unbelievable. I couldn't possibly make this s**t (pun intended) up!

After surgery, I could go three thousand miles before needing a commode and now I couldn't go three blocks. Our romantic getaway consisted of one singular focus: looking for restrooms. I've even learned the word in multiple languages: *salle de bain, baño, seomra folctha, koupelna.* Can you tell how many Los Angeles neighborhoods I had been in that day?

As I was dreaming about (and using!) restrooms all day long, I wondered what ever happened to the old expression "in by nine, out by five"? Now, for me, it was "in at nine, out *in* five—*if I was lucky.*"

You would be amazed at how undiscerning you become when you really have to go. A good (or even decent) flush was the only requirement, though I did rate them, with a particular department store earning five stars and a gas station off the 405-101 freeway interchange earning negative-three stars.

One of my favorites was when I asked for the closest (emphasizing *closest*) restroom and received the following response: "Leave out the back door, take a left, then a right, and then go up a ramp and down a long hallway. It will be on your right. You can't miss it." *Huh?* You have to be kidding me, I thought. I was not looking to circumnavigate the globe. Obviously, these people did not see the sweat on my brow or my trembling hands. I had no time, though, to debate these instructions. I just had to hope that I

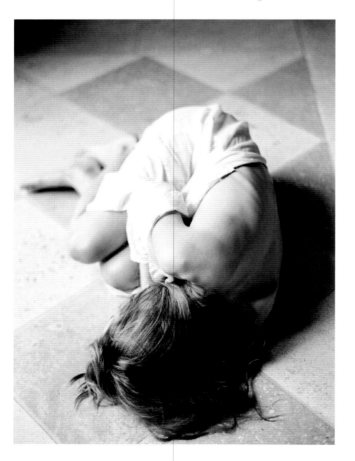

could remember the ludicrous directions and make it in time.

By the early evening, we made it to our hotel. Not exactly the romantic getaway that we had hoped it would be. In fact, I spent the entire night on the floor of the hotel bathroom. A Silver Lining of this ridiculous image is that I was at a nice hotel, on a nice floor.

As a nurse, I knew that I had moved from pesky, annoying, and beleaguering trots and stomach cramping to something altogether different and more serious. I had not kept any food in my system for a full four days. I was watching the weight fall off, which under normal circumstances would have been cause for a happy dance, but in this case, this much weight loss was *not good*. I was starting to get dizzy (and running into things, as evidenced by a knot on my head). The anti-nausea medications that I had been taking were not working. I now found myself on a slippery slope

(and I am *not* a good skier!) and needed a lifeline.

I called my oncologist, who told me that he wanted to intervene—right away. In the meantime, he had me start drinking Gatorade in an attempt to replenish some of the lost electrolytes. However, within ten minutes of my drinking it, the runs came running back. Really? Oh yes, really.

Fast-forward four hours (the time it took to get home, from LA to Santa Barbara, including potty stops) and I found myself at the clinic connected to an IV machine running a liter of fluids into my PORT-A-CATH to offset the dehydration resulting from days on end in the bathroom(s) and to break the diarrhea cycle.

One of the unpleasant side effects of Taxotere is colitis, an inflammatory process in the bowels resulting in diarrhea-diarrhea-diarrhea. With fluids going into my body, my doctor and I put some goals in place, which was good because I am an action-oriented, to-do-list kind of girl:

1. Get me home feeling human. (I felt the need to have that word defined, because those days, I forgot what it meant.)
2. Replenish electrolytes. The fastest, most efficient way for me at the time was by drinking Gatorade.
3. Once drinking had been reintroduced, next on the agenda was to eat, beginning with bananas and then moving on to rice, toast, and even some applesauce.

A Silver Lining of this explosive colitis experience was that I had a Bondurant-trained designated driver (the HOTY) who rose to the occasion and stopped at nothing (and I mean *nothing*) to ensure that I made every pit stop in a timely, accident-free manner. Another Silver Lining was that for a brief moment in time, I knew what it felt like to be model sample size. Let me just say that it ain't worth getting there!

MOUTH MESHUGAAS

The next side effect that I experienced was mucositis, aka mouth sores. I'm not kidding. I wish I were, but I'm not. Three months earlier, even if I had tried really, really hard, I could never have imagined my life changing so abruptly and so radically. At this point, I had been bombed by seemingly all things breast cancer so far.

In case you are unfamiliar (why on earth *would* you be familiar?), cancer-related mouth sores are one of the most common side effects of chemotherapy. I knew that I might see them at some point, but not after the *first* treatment. To clarify, "meshugaas" is a Yiddish word that means "crazy or senseless behavior." These mouth sores were definitely crazy and senseless.

Mouth sores or ulcers (as in open wound) form on the ultrasensitive inside lining of the mouth (mucous membranes) or on the lips (mine were both in my mouth *and* on my lips, of course). Now, these nasty things can extend into the esophagus, which carries food to the stomach.

Why? you ask. Well, the goal of chemotherapy is to kill rapidly growing cancer cells, right? Here's the thing: there are lots of healthy cells in the body that also divide and grow rapidly, including the cells that line the inside of the mouth and hair follicles. Killing them leads to mouth meshugaas and baldness.

My mouthful of mouth sores appeared overnight, and it felt as if the inside of my mouth had been burned. Sorry about that image, but that's what it felt like. They made eating, talking, swallowing, and breathing difficult.

Chemo-related mouth sores tend to be episodic, appearing three to ten days after a chemo treatment. Mine were right on time. Punctuality has always been a strong suit of mine. I was hoping to miss the arrival date for mouth sores, though.

These types of mouth sores usually clear up within a week or so, unless malnutrition slows recovery. The every-five-minute toilet-seeking GI distress probably wasn't conducive to good nutrition, right?

The other kicker: damage to the cells in the mouth makes it difficult for the mouth to heal itself and to fend off germs, leading to the potential for perpetual sores and infections. In other words, there was the possibility for this meshugaas to stick around. There are all kinds of suggestions to get rid of mouth sores. Let's begin with good oral care, such as brushing regularly, preferably after every meal. Also, drink lots of water, keep your mouth moist, and avoid mouthwashes, especially those containing alcohol.

Because of all the digestive issues I was having, my oncologist referred me to the team's dietitian who suggest a number of things:

1. Eat as much nutrient-dense food as you can manage because vitamin deficiencies can make symptoms worse.
2. Avoid spicy and/or salty foods or foods with citric acid or tomato juice. *As if I could eat spicy food!*
3. Avoid foods that are sharp, such as crackers, toast, and dry cereal. *Duh.*
4. Try adding moist foods over dry foods, such as by using gravy and sauces. Good food choices can include mashed potatoes, cooked cereals, applesauce, cottage cheese, pudding, yogurt, smoothies (without citrus), soups, Jell-O, baby food, or food pureed in the blender. How's that for motivating? Delish.
5. Avoid foods with extreme temperatures.
6. In addition to all of these superfun activities to add to my already full breast cancer to-do list, I had to take (by take, I mean "swish and spit") the following medications: magic mouthwash and Lidocaine.

Let's start with magic mouthwash. Yes, that is its real name. I know. I know. I couldn't have made it up if I tried. The outside of the bottle said *red, raspberry, elixir.* Let me just tell you that this phrase equates to *disgusting*. You can't believe how awful this "magical" mouth medicine tasted, at least to me.

In addition to the magic mouthwash, I also took Lidocaine to numb the mouth sores enough so that I could eat. Oh, that's right, because eating is something that I really, really, really wanted to do after the week I had. However, as you may remember, malnutrition encourages mouth sores to hang around, so I *had* to eat. The Lidocaine was a thick, syrupy fluid that I could either apply to my finger and then rub on the sores, or "swish and spit" to get to the mouth sores that were loitering in the back of my mouth. Yes, they popped up everywhere. When the pharmacist suggested that I dilute the Lidocaine because of its strength, I reminded her that horse tranquilizers didn't work on me, so I would be swishing and spitting sans dilution.

The outside of the Lidocaine bottle described the taste as cherry. I'd like to know who in their right mind described this as "cherry." Cherries are good. Delish. Yummy. I love cherries. This was so *not* the taste of cherry. Why couldn't they just say "This is really going to taste terrible, but it will help your mouth sores, so just do it"?

Also on the outside of the bottle was the suggestion about not drinking alcohol while taking Lidocaine. Now, I found that to be just plain mean. While I wished for a supersize glass of chardonnay, I wasn't about to drink during treatment.

A big Silver Lining of this new episode was that the medicines, though completely vile tasting, did work. My mouth was fully numb (and I slurred as if I were three sheets to the wind!), which eliminated the overt pain and enabled me to eat a little more.

A VERY (UN)HAIRY SITUATION

Because I seemed to be the poster child for chemo side effects (i.e., *all* of them), it didn't come as a complete shock to me that hair loss was next on the list. It was the second (or maybe the third or fourth) shoe to drop. For three years before my diagnosis, I wore my hair short, really short. I used to have long hair (all one length, past my shoulders). However, between blowouts, straightening treatments, updos, and split ends, maintaining it became annoying. So I went with a pixie cut.

Fast-forward to breast cancer baldness. Being bald-bald-bald was, I knew, inevitable. Hair loss occurs because, as you may recall, chemotherapy

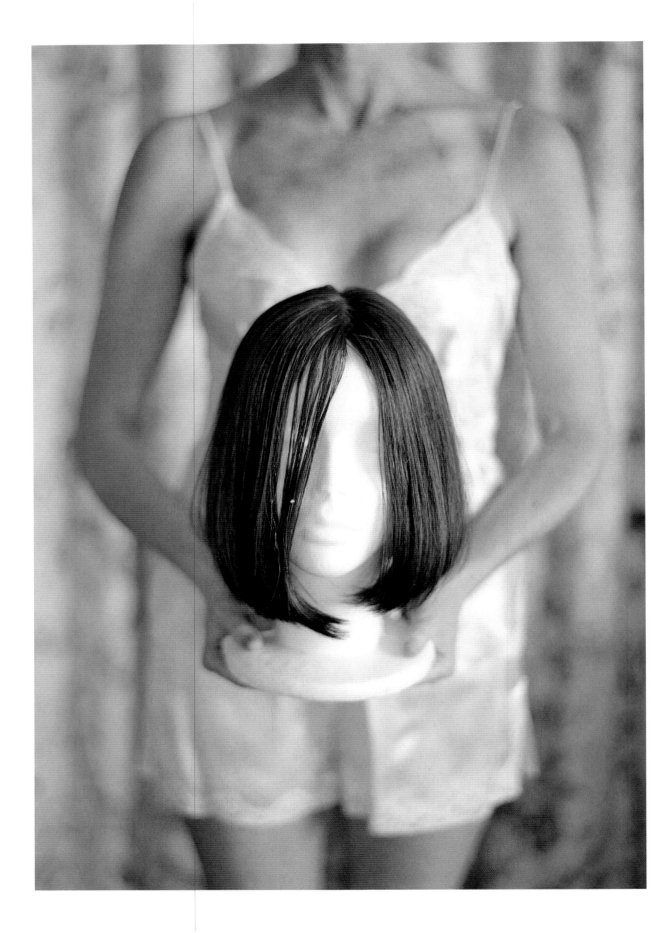

targets all rapidly dividing cells—healthy cells as well as cancer cells. First the rapidly dividing cells in my mouth and now the rapidly dividing cells on my head and yes, elsewhere.

Two weeks after my first dose of chemo, my head felt prickly and itchy, which, I assumed, was the precursor to hair loss (*bingo!*). The best way to describe the feeling is as if I had worn a hat all day, from morning until night, then took it off and needed a really good rub to get rid of the prickles and itches.

In addition to the prickles and itches, I had clumps of hair coming out in my hand. Big clumps with absolutely no pattern whatsoever. *Ewwww.* So, with this unsolicited outpouring of hair follicles, I knew it was time to shave my head. I chose to shave my head for the following reasons (which also happened to be Silver Linings):

1. To give me a sense of control. Breast cancer was causing this, but I could do something about it.
2. To get rid of the prickly, itchy feeling.

I have to admit that, despite my planning and sense of control, I was surprisingly nervous about it. Again, I was entering a foreign, unknown territory. However, an amazing girlfriend lovingly planned the entire event. Using the word "event" may sound a little dramatic. Well, the reality is that it *is* dramatic to shave your head because you have to take *chemotherapy*.

Anyway, she asked the owner of a local barbershop (whom I had never met) whether he would stay open late to shave my head in a private atmosphere. Ah, what a gift. My girlfriend planned everything, but I did have one rule for the evening: no crying. I wanted to focus on the absurdity of the entire situation and find Silver Linings in the form of humor while doing the deed.

My barber was the most amazing man imaginable. He was kind, gentle, thoughtful, sensitive, and he had a fabulous sense of humor! The added bonus was that he had done chemo coiffure before, which was incredibly comforting. One of the first things he told me was that prior

to my arrival he sterilized all of his equipment so that I need not worry about any problems or infections. How thoughtful and sensitive (and smart!) was that?

Before he started, I asked him whether he would give me a Mohawk (I had secretly always wanted to see myself in a Mohawk). Why? Heaven only knows—perhaps to add a little humor to the situation? Or maybe it was because I spent my adolescence in the middle of Indiana during the eighties, when seemingly everyone (including boyfriends one, two, and three) had Mohawks. He just chuckled and said, "Sure, whatever you want." To Mohawkville I went.

Buzzzzzzzz. Oh my goodness, did we ever laugh. It was the first time I had laughed— really laughed—since I began treatment. It felt so incredibly good.

When the deed was done and I was bald, I realized, as is the case with everything in life, that the anticipation was far worse than the reality. I shaved my head and now it was bald. It was as simple as that. I put on my new wig (which the HOTY and I picked out on the colitis tour of LA) and was ready to walk out into the world.

While I didn't quite feel like "bald is beautiful" (on me), I did leave the barbershop feeling that "bald ain't so bad."

> ### LIFELINE
>
> *Your bald head will get cold. Invest in a soft cap. It's worth it. Your head will get hot. Don't use an ice cap because it will only make your head feel as if it's stuck in the freezer.*

FOREWARNED IS FOREARMED

Prior to the second round of chemo, the HOTY and I had a talk with my oncologist about how to aggressively treat chemo side effects prophylactically, *before* they descended again! He told me that I essentially had had every side effect imaginable. In other words, we knew how (badly!) my body reacted to chemotherapy, so our philosophy became "forewarned is forearmed."

So, the day after chemo, since I was going in for my Neulasta shot anyway, he planned to give me IV fluids to (hopefully!) help prevent some of the outrageous nausea that I had. Additionally, after the first infusion of chemo, mouth sores surfaced on day eight, so to hopefully prevent them, I started using the magic mouthwash (that name still blows my mind) on day seven. The goal was to outsmart the side effects.

> ### LIFELINE
>
> *I was an anomaly when it came to side effects. Most people do not have nearly the extent or the intensity of the side effects that I encountered!*

According to my oncologist, I had seen the worst of the worst side effects, so by that point, we knew what we were dealing with. If or when side effects presented themselves, I would be much more prepared and ready to handle them, which was a Silver Lining.

REGURGITAS

Chemo turned me into Puke Face. There's simply no other way to describe it. And the kicker was that I have always *despised* throwing up. In my non–breast cancer life, when I have the stomach flu, I will lie in bed for days rather than toss my cookies. I'm *not* one of those people who believe that retching is cathartic, who feel "better" after.

Not only do I think it's abhorrent, but I am so unattractive when I heave. I moan, cry, and laugh. Yes, laugh—that nervous, twitchy, screechy laughter. Kind of like people sometimes do at funerals. Ever seen that? I feel so sorry for those people, as I do for myself when I upchuck.

Here's an example of how my Puke Face interfered with my life. One day, when I was feeling relatively human ("relative" being the operative word) the HOTY and I planned to go on a lunch date, which was a heartwarming idea. I was craving yummy fish tacos (the clean,

healthy, non-fried variety) from one of my favorite restaurants. So, we put the convertible top down and cruised in the sunshine (I was wearing a hat and doused in sunscreen of course).

On the drive, he asked me a couple of questions about my day (in the interest of good marital communication) and I found that I couldn't talk—because I was so nauseous.

I told him that I needed to reschedule our date and just go home (I was not the ideal date—*again!*). On the way home, it (meaning the immediate urge to heave) hit me like a Mack truck, requiring a *rapid response*. Of course, we were on the 101 highway, eight minutes from our home, doing about seventy miles per hour, when I felt that awful, dreaded sensation in my esophagus (I felt it in my esophagus because I ignored it in my stomach).

All I was able to utter was "Pull over." The HOTY coasted on the side of the road for what seemed like an eternity (though I'm sure he would beg to differ, citing the reality that it was a mere handful of seconds) and then I said "*Noooooooowwwww!*" at which time he stopped immediately. I then proceeded to open the door and get my head out quickly enough to empty the contents of my stomach. The HOTY was amazing, handing me a towel and water and patting my head.

After I was done, with tears, snot, and drool still pouring out of me, the HOTY said, "If you feel better later, maybe we could go out to dinner." He was serious. Really?

Really? I felt so sad for him. All he wanted to do was go out to lunch and have a nice conversation. That's all.

The Silver Linings of that particular day (because you *know* I had to find some!):

1. Gratitude for being married to the kindest, most sensitive and loving HOTY—ever.
2. I made it to the side of the road, in a stopped car. Thank goodness because highway regurgitas presents a unique problem: BRDS (Barf Return Due to Speed).

SCARF STARES

After a few days, I had come to accept my bald head. Every time something was taken away from me (my breasts, my hair, my dignity), I felt more grateful for what I still did have, such as a positive attitude. Silver Linings could never be taken away from me.

Even though I had a wig that was made out of real hair and was actually fairly attractive, it was still uncomfortable and itchy. I found that I really only wanted to wear it for short periods of time (such as when taking our daughter to preschool or going out on the rare evening). Scarves were simply much more comfortable.

> **LIFELINE**
>
> *Cotton scarves are easiest to tie & most effective at staying on your head.*

I invested in some really chic cotton ones that tied easily, didn't slip, and were very lightweight. After playing around with them and finding my "look," I felt pretty good.

What unexpectedly descended on me were the Scarf Stares. Whoa. They came out of nowhere. The first time I really noticed them I was feeling pretty put together in my floral scarf, sparkly earrings, and coordinating outfit. I had to go get my blood drawn before my second round of chemo. While in the waiting room, a woman (who had to be in her mid-sixties) was sitting across from me, staring—full-on staring. She made absolutely no attempt to divert her stare. It was so outrageously overt that I finally just had to call her out.

"Can I help you with something, ma'am?" I asked.

She looked horrified. "N-n-n-no," she said.

"Why are you staring at me, then?"

"I don't know," she said.

"Well, if you want to talk about something, please do let me know," I said.

Geez Louise, those steroids made me do and say things that pre—breast cancer I never would have imagined. However, she really should have known better, right? I'm now all too aware that most people don't, in fact, know better.

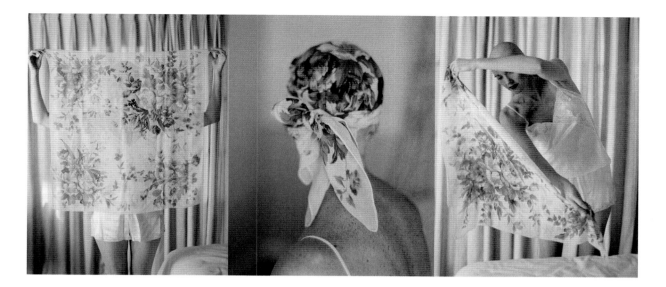

I was in the clinic a few days later, getting fluids, when a young woman came in with her mother. I overheard her (the daughter, not the mother) say that she was getting her Neulasta shot. Wow, I thought. Here was another young woman with breast cancer. She had a full head of hair, leading me to believe that she had just had her first round of chemo.

I was sitting in my treatment chair and when I looked up, both mother and daughter were staring right at me. I smiled. I understood why they were staring. This was so unlike the previous situation. In this circumstance, I had complete empathy, knowing that they were staring because the young woman knew that she too would soon be bald. I simply smiled at her with an "It will be okay" look.

What I came to realize was that there would simply be a whole lot of staring for a few months. Most of the time, the stares were filled with sympathy. They really didn't make me feel any better, but I knew it was not about me. Seeing me may have reminded them of a friend or loved one with cancer. Seeing me may just have made them sad that there is so much cancer in the world. I don't really know. I just kept my head high and tried to go on about my days.

HELLACIOUS HOTNESS HITS

Lots of people (too many, in fact) asked, "Have you had any hot flashes . . . *yet*?" There was a little part of me (okay, a big part of me) who wanted to jump up and down and say: "No . . . Not yet!! Maybe, just maybe, I won't get them!!"

Though I knew it was only a matter of time (because the type of chemotherapy for women with estrogen-positive breast cancer hastens the onset of menopause and subsequently produces hot flashes), I held out hope that I might actually avoid one side effect of chemo: hellacious hot flashes. Nice try. I can just imagine the chemo saying: "*Na-na-na-na-naaaaaah-na!*"

When the hot flashes started, I didn't exactly know what they were. I woke up, looked around our room, listened to the HOTY snore, tapped my feet, counted sheep, and hoped for sleep. Then, I noticed that I felt really warm. Did the HOTY crank up the heat? I wondered. Geesh, I was *hot*. I took off my little skullcap that I wore every night to keep my bald head warm, but I was still hot. Then I shed my pajama top so that I was laying in my tank top. What on earth was going on? I managed to go back to sleep (sort of dozed, actually) and didn't think much of it. Denial? Probably.

Now, these were not the sweats of the sacred sweat lodge variety originated by the Native Americans (which include guided prayer, chanting, drumming, and spiritual cleanliness). This was more like: "OMG, I'm on *fire*. Call 9-1-1 . . . *noooooow!*"

In the meantime, off came the tank top (I was officially naked from the waist up!), socks, blanket . . . As soon as I was stripped down, things turned cold. In an instant I felt as if I had been dunked in an ice bath. Was it possible (how could it be?) that I was now having a cold flash? I was as confused as I was cold. Back on with the cap, pajama top, socks, and blanket . . . and the shivering started. Oh, and I was wide awake. Good times.

LIFELINE

Talk with your doctor about possible ways to help relieve hot flashes. There are lots of options. Just because they didn't work for me doesn't mean that they won't work for you!

From that point on, I was crowned the Hot Flash Queen, earning the title by having four to five ginormous hot flashes every hour, twenty-four hours a day. There are lots of (nonhormonal) things to try to help diminish the intensity and frequency of hot flashes (e.g., vitamin E, vitamin B6, Effexor), but nothing did the trick for me (that's not to say it won't work for you, though!). What helped me was wearing layers and carrying a fan with me 24/7 for the next nine months. Literally.

NOT FIGHTING

Omnipresent in our culture are cancer "fighting" messages, as in "cancer-fighting strategies" and "cancer-fighting foods" and "cancer-fighting treatments." After my breast cancer diagnosis, I found myself cringing when people referred to me as a "fighter" or suggest that I "keep fighting." Midway through treatment, I decided that fighting was not something I wanted to do. Most people assumed that my outrageous philosophy was a by-product of chemotherapy or pain meds or just the general delirium that comes with a cancer diagnosis.

Was treatment awful? Yes. Was it a struggle? Of course. Did it rock me to my core? Absolutely. However, I still fervently believe that I never engaged in a fight with breast cancer.

Frankly, the thought of "fighting" made my stomach turn because, quite simply, I'm not a fighter. Now, that's certainly not to say that I'm passive. Far, far from it. In fact, the image of myself as passive makes me laugh out loud. I'm assertive. Strong. Determined. Forthright.

I know quite a few people who are "fighters." They love to pick a fight and then go full throttle: yelling and screaming with smoke coming out of their ears. These are the people who, when you look at them, seem as if they are seething, just waiting for the next battle. I have never in my life understood how someone could live this way.

If I haven't thrown you over the edge and you are still reading, please allow me to clarify that fighting is very different from the emotion of anger. Anger is, I believe, a very healthy emotion. When I'm really ticked about something (which does happen on occasion), I acknowledge it, welcome it, process it, and then politely ask it to leave. Anger isn't something that I'm fond of holding for long periods of time.

So, if I didn't "fight," are you wondering what on *earth* I did during the year of my treatment? Well, let me tell you that there are tons of *positive* things that I did during treatment: I harnessed energy. I looked for inspiration and encouragement in the form of Silver Linings. I laughed (at myself, mostly). I rested. I gave the treatments the time and space they needed to eradicate cancer from my body. I learned and grew. I tried things that I had never done before (e.g., giving myself IV fluids, tying a scarf on a—my—bald head, photography, writing, qigong). I allowed people to care for and love me. Fighting, to me, has a tremendously pejorative connotation. Why add insult (fighting) to injury (cancer)? During treatment, my philosophy was to focus on the positive and thereby render the negative inconsequential.

Here's another thing: in all of my years as a cardiac nurse, never once did we (nurses, doctors, other health care professionals) tell patients with cardiovascular disease to "fight." Why, I wonder, are people with cancer the only patients who are told to "fight"? Why "fight" cancer but not heart disease. I've never understood this.

As a hospice nurse who cared for many cancer patients at the end of their lives, I wondered whether they were somehow to blame because they "lost the fight." It seemed almost punitive to suggest that they "lost." As if they had something to do with it. It was never suggested that patients with cardiac disease, for example, "lost" some kind of "battle."

There is certainly no right or wrong here. Each person chooses how she will handle her own circumstances and disease process. As a matter of fact, one of my dearest friends who was diagnosed with a different type of cancer chose the fighting analogy to give her strength. My fundamental hope is that no matter which approach you choose, you are able to find Silver Linings (inside the ring or out).

CHEMO SOBBY

The week after the third round was really rough. It knocked me down—*hard*. The cumulative effect of three doses of TAC chemotherapy took its toll physically, mentally, and emotionally. It was during this period that I met a new companion: Chemo Sobby. Thanks to Chemo Sobby, I cried at the drop of a hat. Literally.

One evening, the HOTY went to a party that I really wanted to attend but couldn't possibly attend because I was too sick. To add insult to my already hare-brained situation, the Young Dubliners, one of our favorite Irish bands, were play-

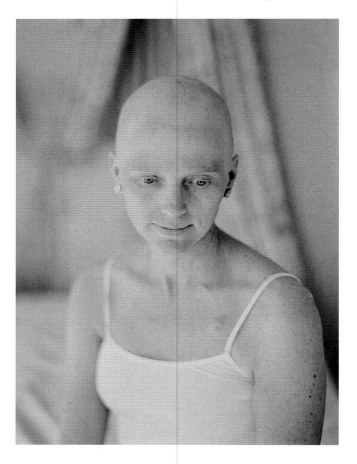

ing. While the HOTY was out and Lalee was sleeping, I couldn't focus on a thing. Not a book, movie, or magazine. All I was left with were the thoughts in my mushy, overwrought, absent-minded brain combined with a series of hot flashes as regular and (for me, as uncomfortable) as labor contractions. At some point, the HOTY texted (un-doubtedly with the Young Dubliners playing in the background): "You okay? Want me to come home?"

Of course I wanted him to come home and wallow in my misery. Of course I wanted him to be with me as I writhed in the discomfort of my relentless bone pain. Of course I wanted him to rub my feet and tell me everything was going to be okay. Fortunately, though, I held my neuroses hostage and told him to stay and have a good time. By eleven o'clock, however, I was a complete wreck, having moved from our bedroom to the family room to seek cooler pastures and a darkness that I hoped would keep my mental maladjustment at bay.

When he rolled in, I must have been quite a sight: wearing a skullcap down to my nose, scarf quadruple-wrapped around my neck, and flannel snowman pajamas with the pants pulled up over my knees. To add to the übersexy look, my arms and legs were spread à la the Nestea Plunge commercials circa 1978. When he came in and saw me, he chuckled (justifiably!). Well, well, well, that little chuckle, that tiny little laugh let the wild, untamed Chemo Sobby loose. I went into a wailing fit of tears, the likes of which frightened even me. I said, "Why are you laughing at me? How could you laugh at me?"

With that question, I put the poor guy in an impossible position. I mean, really, don't you feel for him? What on earth does one say to that? He was forced to lie (we both knew he was lying) and say, "I'm not laughing at you, honey." Then he promptly exited the room and went to the kitchen for a piece of chocolate. He came back a few minutes later and asked whether he could help me get to bed (not to sleep, mind you, but to bed).

The only thing that stopped me from crying was the threat of losing more eyelashes, which, my friends, was a highly motivating factor! Did I forget to tell you that you lose the hair not only on your head but also *everywhere* else? Sorry about that. Yes, you lose your eyebrows, eyelashes, underarm hair, and, yes, even *there.* I felt like a prepubescent child. There were times, as a bald skeleton, when I felt as if I had lost every last shred of dignity.

The HOTY proceeded to tuck me in, kiss me on the forehead, and tell me how much he loved me. Can you imagine? All that love *after* my Chemo Sobbing. Do you see why he is the HOTY and my ultimate Silver Lining?

> **LIFELINE**
>
> *My BFF, LiFT, was a constant source of strength & inspiration. When things were as bad as they could be, I could call her, compare notes & kvetch. If you can, find a mentor who has had breast cancer (& similar treatments) to be your lifeline to help you get through treatment.*

OTHER SIDE EFFECTS

In addition to the biggies, I also had quite a few other side effects to add to my (dirty) laundry list. These included, in no order of importance, priority, or drama:

NAIL CHANGES: I had no idea what this meant in the little pamphlet I was given before chemo started. What it meant for me was that not only would they stop growing and become soft and mushy, but they also would develop grooves that would take nearly a year to disappear after treatment ended. Supersexy.

DRY SKIN: Dry as in "Am I *molting*?" I applied and reapplied moisturizer all day long, which did help (Silver Lining).

CHANGE IN TASTE BUDS: This was a unique experience for me because I love food. The loss of flavor added insult to injury.

RUNNY NOSE: You also lose the hair in your *nose,* which meant that I dripped like a leaky faucet 24/7. The Silver Lining was that my girlfriend gave me the most beautiful linen hankies with my monogram, which made me feel a wee bit feminine.

DECREASED LIBIDO: This was the understatement of the year. I mean, really. Can you just imagine anything less sexy than being a bald, hairless skeleton?

While I continued to look for and always found Silver Linings in every day, I don't want to give the impression that, for one second, any of this was easy-breezy. Having breast cancer is stunningly hard. The side effects were horrendous. I literally felt like a Puke Face every minute of every day. I was in a persistent, foggy state of forgetfulness. I didn't sleep with any efficacy and I felt like I had a jackhammer in the middle of my bones.

Despite all of this, yes, I maintained a Silver Lined attitude. Silver Linings consistently, and often persistently, gave me balance and perspective. Happiness, I now know, is an attitude, a choice. I stayed true to the decision that I made at the time of my diagnosis that no amount of pain or breast cancer misery in the world could take away my spirit.

THE LIGHT AT THE END OF THE CHEMO DESPAIR TUNNEL

On the day that I was supposed to have my fifth of six chemo infusions, I had not yet recovered from the last round of chemo (three whole weeks prior!). As a consequence, my oncologist and I decided (everything was a joint decision with him!) that I needed another week to recover. I have to tell you that it was kind of like a snow day from school (on a day with an *exam*!). You know that feeling of being released from a pressure-filled obligation—knowing in the back of your mind that it wasn't gone for good—but relishing in the wide-open freedom? Well, that's how I felt!

In addition to delaying chemo, because of my inability to recover, we changed the remainder of my chemotherapy regimen altogether, with the goal of making life livable while continuing to eradicate breast cancer.

Changing a patient's chemotherapy regimen is not done very often. It's not an ideal situation, though it's not the end of the world. Generally, the way to think about it is that if a person has "standard, frequently seen breast cancer" (i.e., nothing particularly rare), then standard chemo regimens are used. If that person (like myself) reacts poorly (I'm clearly *under*exaggerating here), then a custom regimen is created.

The truth of the matter is that, like I said before, medicine is as much of an art as it is a science. Each of us is unique and, therefore, we react very differently to all kinds of things, not the least of which is chemotherapy.

So, we eliminated Taxotere because my oncologist believed that this was the drug that was responsible for most of my severe problems, and we replaced it with Taxol (which is in the same class of drugs, kind of like a cousin) and added *one* more dose (instead of two) of Adriamycin combined with Cytoxan.

> ### LIFELINE
> *When you're on the art side of medicine, it is important to be open, flexible, &, yes, creative.*

Why, you ask, did we not start with this plan originally? Well, so much of decision making depends on the clinical data (i.e., research) that support a choice. All clinical data (pathology reports, margins, size of tumors, etc.) pointed my treatment plan to Taxotere. However, we learned that my body was too sensitive to the Taxotere. Therefore, we switched to Taxol, which is in the same class of drugs but is less toxic. Taxol has side effects that are comparable to Taxotere's, but less severe and intense.

My favorite Silver Lining of this plan was that I no longer had to take the steroids. I had taken them to offset (supposedly) the side effects of the Taxotere. The steroids were horrendous, absolutely awful. I actually came to dread their side effects as much as I dreaded the chemo itself.

Another Silver Lining to the change of plans was that (with the exception of seizures) I had already had every single side effect. Why was this a Silver Lining? Well, because I knew what to expect. The ability to prepare for side effects was very helpful in coping with them. Most people say, "Oh, no one has *all* of the side effects." Well, I'm here to prove those naysayers wrong.

> ### LIFELINE
> *Being able to prepare for side effects can be empowering. If your side effects are as bad as mine were (I sure hope not!), do whatever it takes to create the time & space to allow your body to heal.*

As I've said earlier, my philosophy in life, and certainly during this mess, is to hope for the best and prepare for the worst. So I found myself hoping and preparing. My oncologist hoped that with the lower dose of Taxol given more frequently (every week), the side effects would at least be mitigated. Hoping. Again.

After I left the appointment with my oncologist, tears of relief and joy streamed down my face. I saw this as a major turning point in this treatment process. I envisioned myself regaining a certain semblance of my life. I was over-the-moon thrilled!

A week later, I was back in my chemo chair for my last dose of Adriamycin and Cytoxan and my first dose of Taxol. As I always did before chemo, I looked at it, welcomed it into my body, and expressed gratitude for it. I appreciated all that it did to get rid of breast cancer in my body. This gratitude led to more gratitude. There were a lot of sick people in the clinic that day. I do know this sounds odd. All of the patients were ill, obviously. But there is sick and there is SICK. And you know what one of the SICK people talked about? Attitude. He talked about how attitude makes all of the difference. How's that for a whopping Silver Lining?

Yet another Silver Lining of that day was that I had my *last doses* of Adriamycin and Cytoxan—*ever* (I hope). I was really glad that it was my last dose of Adriamycin, because its most toxic side effect is life-threatening heart damage.

On a side note, I forgot that the red color of Adriamycin passes through the kidneys and, um, produces an unsettling color in the toilet after you drink a lot of water. Catch my drift? This happened to startle me, which then made my heart skip a beat, which then made me think that I was having a cardiac reaction! No worries, though. It was evidence that my kidneys were working just fine. Phew.

The few days after this dose of chemo were as tough and miserable as every other dose. For the first time since my diagnosis, I was *mad*. Lalee had a *Wizard of Oz* performance that I could not attend because I was a *Vomitosaurus rex,* lying on the floor of my bathroom with Chemo Sobby at my side. To barf on the side of the 101 freeway with the HOTY was one thing. Yes, that was pathetic. And gross. But today, to miss Lalee's performance (for which we had been practicing for weeks) made me stratospherically angry. To top it off, when she came home, the first thing she said was, "How are you, Mommy? Is your tummy better? Don't be sorry for missing my performance. I just want you to feel better." Even though she tried so hard to make me feel better, I felt *worse*.

I was also just plain mad that she had to deal with breast cancer in her young life. Was she coping? Yes. Was she as well adjusted as she could be? Yes. Neither of these ameliorated my anger at the fact that she had to deal with this.

ENOUGH

It was at this point that my body and mind were screaming at me: "Enough! Done! Finished! No more!" As I was lying in various positions on the bathroom floor (because I couldn't get the five feet to my bed), I kept wondering, "How much chemo is enough? At what point does the toxicity cease to be effective and start to cause harmful long-term ramifications? When does my body get to have a say in the treatment plan?"

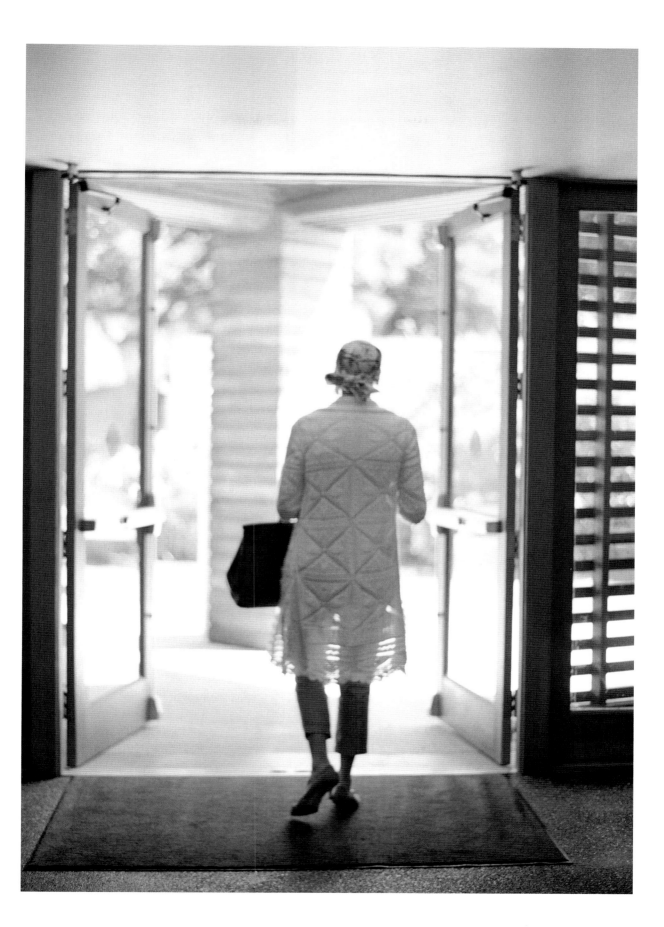

These were certainly rhetorical questions, considering the fact that my sole goal of the day was to get off my bathroom floor and avoid dehydration. I now found myself at a real crossroads, with big decisions to make about chemo and radiation: To do. Not to do. If doing, how much? Rather than make my breast cancer situation subjective (as Chemo Sobby was wont to do), I needed to be fully objective as I planned the next steps in revising my plan of care. The HOTY and I made an appointment to talk with my oncologist about where we were to go from here.

My oncologist came up with a proposition: one more dose of Taxol with as much hydration (to offset the side effects) as possible. I looked at him with glassy eyes and a blank stare. Reactionless. Emotionless. I was neither happy nor sad and no longer mad. It was the HOTY who asked about the cost-benefit analysis of this dose.

"There is no mathematical answer to determine the marginal benefit of the dose," my oncologist said.

"The closer to the end of the plan, the less likely any more chemo makes a real difference," he said.

"There are not enough subtraction studies (i.e., research related to reducing the number of doses of chemo given) demonstrating the outcome," he said.

"The reason for making the effort to explore the possibility of doing more Taxol is because of your (young!) age. However, there is no definitive conclusion that Taxol is (or isn't) going to make a significant difference," he said.

In a nutshell, I had now entered a space in which the marginal benefit of chemo could not be measured.

"The point at which we do no harm," he said.

Hearing this was a watershed moment for me in which I realized that more chemo is not necessarily better. Sometimes, more chemo is just that: more chemo. And chemo, by the way (in case you've missed it), is toxic.

Speaking of more is more, I had more side effects the last round of chemo: neuropathy (dysfunction of one or more peripheral nerves) so bad that I couldn't feel any of my fingertips or toes. The best way to describe the feeling (or lack thereof) is that it was as if I had put my fingers and toes into bowls of ice . . . for about three hours. And they stayed frozen. Taking a shower actually hurt them. Thank you, Taxol.

Back to our dialogue with my oncologist, who said that while there are no data supporting the discontinuation of chemotherapy, after all of these years, he can look at a patient, see the blank stare, and just know. He described it as "the stare that says, 'When does the war end and when is the camp liberated?' " Apparently the stare that I gave him earlier was that stare.

The HOTY and I found ourselves wondering, "How do we know if we're making the right decision? If I don't get the last doses of Taxol in, will breast cancer come back? If so, when and where?" My oncologist gave one succinct, comprehensive, and calming answer to all of these questions when he said, "You do what you can do and then you don't look back. Ever. There was a chance that you were cured the day we met [after my surgery]. We are going to be confident that you are cured as a result of all of the chemo that you have done."

This was an opportunity to remind myself of what I did do, not what I didn't do. After all, I had four rounds of TAC (Taxotere, Adriamycin, and Cytoxan), one round of AC (Adriamycin and Cytoxan), and one round of Taxol. That's some heavy-duty, serious, kick-arse (an Irish term) chemotherapy.

Because this was such a big decision, I corroborated everything with another oncologist. Second opinions, by the way, are an absolute necessity when making decisions of this magnitude.

So, after this appointment, I was done with chemo. That was it. No more. Walking out of the clinic that day felt a little anticlimactic. Perhaps I expected bells and whistles and maybe even a gold star? One thing for sure: I breathed a great big sigh of relief and knew that I took as much chemo as my body could handle.

A BIG DAY

Before any big event, my dear, beloved mother-in-law used to say to her boys (and then to her grandchildren), "Today is a big day." The day that I had my PORT-A-CATH removed was indeed a big day. The vehicle through which chemotherapy went for four and a half months was gone, baby gone.

To have it removed, I had to go back to the Interventional Radiology Department at the hospital and climb on the exact same table on which I had it installed. Taking it out involved snipping a couple of sutures that held it in and then yanking the long tube (it felt as if it was eight feet long!). It hurt like nobody's business. But you know what? I was so flippin' happy that there was no way that this physical pain could overtake my emotional joy.

Leaving the hospital PORT-A-CATH free, I felt such an incredible sense of success, triumph, and completion. Being done—completely done!—with chemotherapy was a glorious Silver Lining. ♥

THE SILVER LINING

Though chemo took me to the deepest, darkest, most unimaginable places, I found **balance**, **perspective**, and **strength** in the form of Silver Linings. On my hardest days, a glimmer of **hope** would appear when I least expected it, from watching a hummingbird outside my window (because I was too weak to stand) to receiving a **gift** left in my mailbox to opening a "thinking about you" email. It was the little things that gave me the strength and the **courage to go on** when I didn't think I could endure another moment.

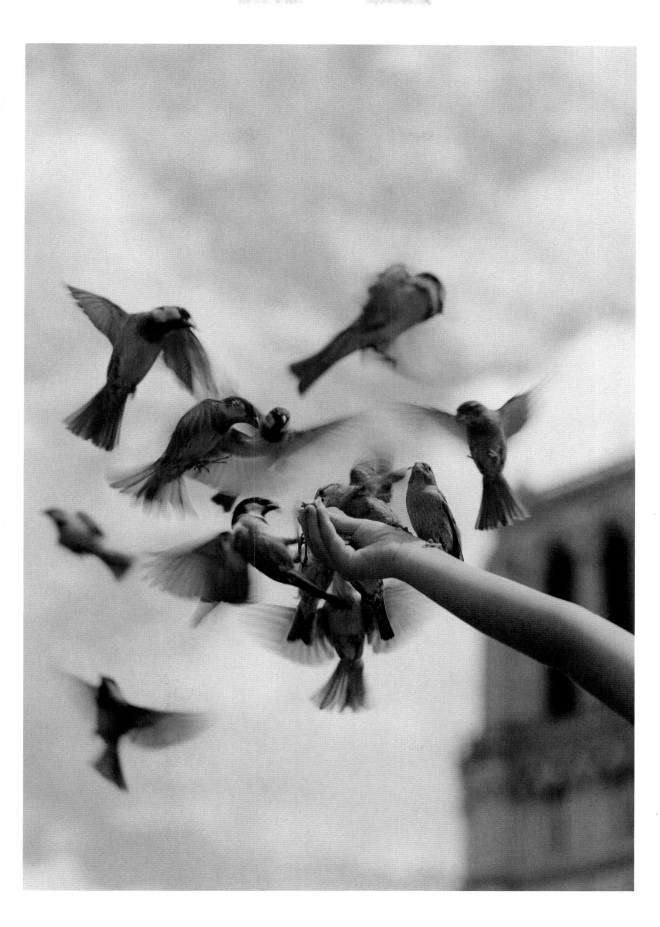

Remember This

- Before beginning chemo, go to the dentist for a checkup and teeth cleaning because you can't do it during chemo.

- Keep a calendar with you at all times to keep track of when you take medications as well as the gazillions of appointments that you will have.

- Keep a journal to record physical side effects. Keeping track of *everything* that happens to you (e.g., nausea, constipation, hot flashes) and when will help your health care team determine whether there are adjustments that can be made to medications to prevent side effects.

- One of the best ways to flush the chemotherapy through your body and out as soon as it has done its job is to drink water. Drink. Drink. Drink.

- Even though you don't have hair, wash and moisturize your scalp at least two times a week.

- Be sure to let your physician know if you have any signs of infection, including fever, change in cough or a new cough, sore throat, shortness of breath, nasal congestion, any redness or swelling, or new onset of pain, to name a few.

- If you start having strange, metallic tastes in your mouth when you eat, use anything *other* than metal utensils.

- Don't shower too much. Because your skin is so dry during chemo, excessive showers strip away moisture.

- I highly recommend touring the treatment room before your first infusion. This way you will know what to expect.

- PORT-A-CATH placement and removal happens in the Interventional Radiology Department of a hospital. Placement can be uncomforatble. Ask for plenty of pain medication.

- If you have a PORT-A-CATH, get an EMLA cream prescription at least one day before chemo. Please learn from my experience!

- You may hear doctors and nurses refer to Ativan as "vitamin A." This is because it is so effective at calming anxiety. Ativan was definitely a Silver Lining during my treatment.

- Know exactly what is expected before your first dose of chemo. It varies from person to person, so ask!

What to Take to Chemo

- Insurance information.
- Any supplements that you are taking.
- Your chemo calendar to record treatments and your response to them.
- A journal to take notes and do some creative writing.
- Entertainment: a phone (and its charger!), iPad, and/or laptop, as well as magazines and a book.
- Clothing: layers, because it can be cold or you could have a hot flash and sizzle.
- Snacks: bland, non-smelly food such as bananas and crackers as well as ginger candies.
- Beverages: water, homemade ginger ale.

Questions to Ask Your Oncology Staff

1. Is Oncotype DX testing right for me?
2. Do I need chemotherapy?
3. What type of chemotherapy will I need?
4. How many drugs?
5. How many cycles?
6. What is the timing for medication delivery?
7. What types of side effects can I expect and when?
8. What types of medications will I take for side effects?
9. Can I work during treatment? How much time will I need to take off?
10. Am I eligible for short- or long-term disability?
11. Will my insurance cover the cost?
12. How can I incorporate complementary medicine?
13. Will I get a PORT-A-CATH?
14. How long will side effects last?
15. Are there any long-term side effects? If so, how will I manage them?
16. How long will it take for my hair to start growing?
17. How best to communicate with you? Phone? Email? After hours?

Ways to Cope with Hot Flashes

- Use an ice pack (or even a bag of frozen peas) on your head and ears.
- Take a cold shower.
- Drink ice water.
- Wear layers (because the heat can turn to cold in an instant!).
- Avoid caffeine, spicy foods, and alcohol (though I hope you are not drinking right now anyway!).
- Sleep on cotton sheets.
- Wear a lightweight cotton scarf or hat.
- Don't take hot showers or hot baths or sit in hot tubs. This one is kind of obvious.
- Carry a fan with you at all times.
- Stick your head in the freezer. Trust me, it feels really good!
- To the best of your ability, avoid stress and relax as much as possible.
- Talk to your physician about supplements.
- Try acupuncture. Many cancer centers offer this or other treatments at no cost.
- Exercise. Restorative yoga and walking were my preferred (and feasible) forms of exercise.

CHAPTER V

Isolation Island

The Emotional Impact of
Cancer Treatment

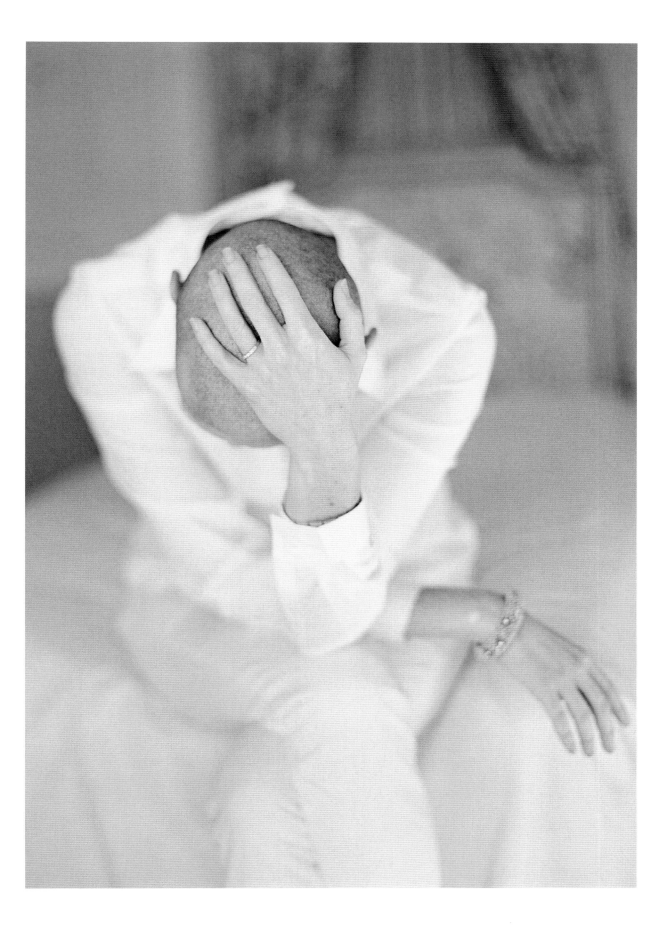

After my fourth round of chemotherapy, I was hospitalized after acquiring an infection with which my nearly nonexistent immune system could not contend. I remember feeling so haggard and beleaguered that I could barely compose myself to put two words together. When I was lying in the hospital bed, it dawned on me that my world seemed to have shrunk, leaving me feeling alone and isolated.

I felt isolated from the most normal and what many people consider to be tedious aspects of life, from school drop-off to work to lunch with friends. I was too sick to go to the grocery store or gym. In other words, I felt isolated from the world. I was living on Isolation Island with Chemo Sobby as my constant companion. Isolation Island isn't a sun-filled place with white sandy beaches and cabana boys at your beck and call. Nope. Not even close. Rather, it more closely resembles a dark, forsaken place in a remote part of Siberia in the middle of winter without any trace of another living creature. (For those who have been, please forgive my understated description.)

There was something about that fourth round of chemo (combined with a hospital stay and returning home with a near 24/7 continuous drip of IV fluids) that made me feel as if I had finally hit the bottom of the cancer treatment barrel. During this period, I had neither the energy nor the capacity to move beyond the confined space that was my bedroom and, eventually, just my bed. Feeling as bad as I did, being around anyone (even my husband and daughter, I'm sad to say) was overwhelming. Now, it wasn't as if friends didn't offer to come over. They did. They offered to sit with me even if I didn't feel like talking. I loved them for that. The most energy that I could muster was to change my IV bag (a Silver Lining of being a nurse-turned-patient).

As a nurse and social worker, I recognized the fact that during extended periods of illness, all sense of time and perspective can fade (and fast!). Illness is an emotionally as well as physically depriving experience. It has the potential to do lasting harm by threatening a person's sense of well-being, competence, and feelings of productivity. Having this professional knowledge is what prevented me from going off the deep end into the breast cancer abyss.

The scope and intensity of these feelings of isolation and subsequent emotional pain fluctuated from day to day. What worried (frightened?) me was that I felt sadder and more distraught than I had ever felt in my life. I was majorly grumpy, easily irritated, and erratically moody. I couldn't

LIFELINE

During prolonged illness, a trip to Isolation Island is normal. The key is preventing it from causing lasting harm.

concentrate. I couldn't sleep despite feeling more exhausted than I had ever been. Ever.

I began to wonder whether the treatment(s) were worse than the disease itself. I literally couldn't bear the thought of another chemo. And I didn't want to leave the house because I was so worried about my persistent nausea and vomiting. I was sick and tired of being a bald, sick person.

The Silver Lining was that these feelings of isolation and despair ultimately carried me closer to invaluable inner resources that I never knew I had. At one point, I refused to be dragged further away from my recognizable self. My incentive for becoming psychologically well was the potential for the future.

What helped me the most was my ability to put on my nurse's cap and assign myself some healthy coping mechanisms, including normalizing and articulating my feelings, slow walks, guided meditation, and restorative yoga. Studies by Bernadine Cimprich at the University of Michigan revealed that the psychological well-being of cancer patients significantly improved after spending twenty minutes a day, three or more days a week, doing restorative activities, including a walk in the woods and gardening.

MARINE LAYER

In Santa Barbara, the summertime usually brings a marine layer of fog that sits over the coast and sometimes the entire city for most of the morning. This same marine layer is present twenty-four hours a day, seven days a week on Isolation Island.

There were many days and even some weeks on end when my cognitive impairment resulting from treatment made me feel as if my brain was literally fogged in. Fatigue, estrogen deficiency, sleep cycle alterations, and depression are all contributing factors to the marine layer on Isolation Island.

A daily occurrence on Isolation Island was attentional fatigue. Yes, this is in addition to physical fatigue. Good times. Attentional fatigue occurs in the face of intense mental effort, when the demands for attention (e.g., when making decisions about treatment) exceed a person's capacity to handle them. Attentional fatigue rendered me utterly useless.

Attentional fatigue ensured that I rarely, if ever, finished something that I started. Reading, cooking, and writing were Herculean tasks. Attentional fatigue can happen at any time from diagnosis through treatment and even into recovery. Mine really hit in the middle of chemotherapy. My mind would wander to the most random and obscure places while trying to complete the most menial of tasks. I'd start to cook something and then go lay down.

> ### LIFELINE
> *Attentional fatigue resulting in decreased concentration is a common occurrence after a cancer diagnosis & during treatment. Even though it makes you feel nuts, you are NOT—I repeat, NOT— losing your mind!*

CRAFT(Y)

Short- and long-term memory loss, or CRAFT (Can't Remember A Flippin' Thing), was an exceptionally debilitating side effect of breast cancer treatment. Being unable to remember the names of people, places, and things made me feel as if my brain was literally turning to mush. It was so bad that one time when I was talking with a friend whom I've known for years, I Could. Not. Remember. Her. Name. The stress of that memory loss then brought on a big hot flash.

Another time, I was driving home and I forgot which freeway exit to take to get to our house. After getting past the shock and awe of not knowing how to get home (*&@%!#$✝!), I took a few deep breaths, pulled over to the side of the road, and put my home address into my car's GPS system. The Silver Lining of the day was that I had GPS!

Prior to my diagnosis, I was the girl who could remember anyone's name after only one meeting. Unfortunately for the HOTY, he came to depend on my masterful ability. However, he quickly learned to stop asking who was who when I just looked at him with an "Are you *kidding* me?" look.

Oh, and one time it took me five tries (okay, eight) to put on Lalee's bathing suit (the kind that has the crisscross in the back). I could not remember for the life of me how to put it on. When Lalee said, "Mommy, you're usually really good at putting on my bathing suit," I nearly burst into tears. The Silver Lining was that I didn't burst into tears and that I eventually got the bathing suit on.

DISORGANIZATION

I have always prided myself on my organization skills. I'm the geeky girl who alphabetizes her books and color-codes her files. I have been in a long-term relationship with a label maker, and last but not least, the clothes in my closet are hung by style, color, and season. *Oh yes, I am that girl.*

Breast cancer laughs in the face of organization. Ha! During treatment, my books and files were piled in top-heavy stacks. The label maker was dusty. And my closet? Piles everywhere.

The thing about disorganization was that it fueled my memory loss and lack of concentration, which then fueled more disorganization. It was a vicious cycle.

To add insult to my disorganized injury, my language skills were altered beyond

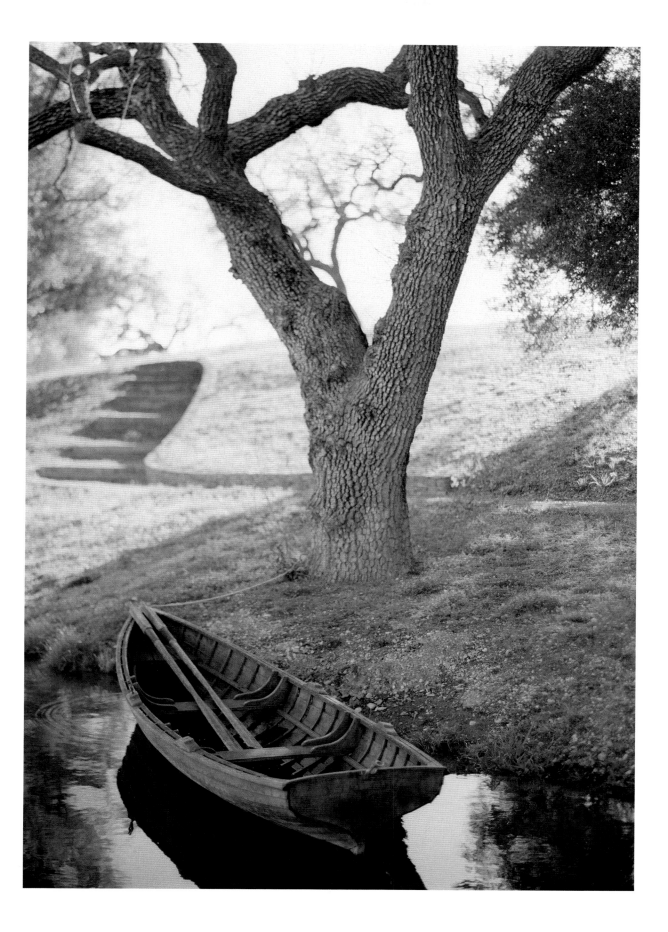

belief. I used to be a good conversationalist, if I do say so myself. But during treatment, words either didn't exist or they floated around in my brain like bubbles that couldn't get out. Either way, I found myself trying to participate in conversations and feeling unable to produce even a single word.

Cognitive impairment was truly the most frightening aspect of breast cancer because it impacted my fundamental abilities to think, problem solve, follow directions, and make decisions. Cognitive ability (or lack thereof) is a huge factor in defining who we are as individuals. Having my cognition altered so radically made me feel incredibly vulnerable.

Now, I'm not telling you all of these things to scare you. Why would I do that? Here's the thing: I wish that I had known about Isolation Island, because when I arrived on it, not knowing where I was or what was happening, I was thrown for a doozy of a loop. Had I known that Isolation Island existed, the experience could have been a tiny bit demystified and perhaps—just perhaps—I could have prepared myself for my stay.

While in this sorry state, I developed coping mechanisms and held on to the belief that words and memory would come back. I clung to the hope that the fatigue would dissipate. And you know what? The ultimate Silver Lining of this pervasively dark and cloudy marine layer in my head and heart was that—just as the sun eventually comes out in the afternoon in Santa Barbara—the sun came out in my head, heart, and soul, slowly at first and then more frequently and consistently.

ROLE REVERSAL

Learning how to rely on people when I was sick was extremely hard for me. As a nurse, mom, and social worker, I had always been the caregiver. And I liked it that way. Until my diagnosis, I had always been a do-it-yourselfer. However, breast cancer had other plans for me because it sucked every bit of my ability to manage even the most meager activities of daily living right out of me.

Not only did I have to accept my own cancer patient role as a dependent, but my family and friends also had new roles to learn. A cancer diagnosis doesn't happen just to you. It also happens to your family, friends, and community. People who were directly or indirectly impacted by my illness—from my husband to my daughter's teacher—sought to identify their roles in my treatment, to figure out what they could contribute to the experience.

Though it took some work, I knew that it was up to me to identify who would do what. For example, one friend organized food delivery (if not for me, then for my family). Another friend was the designated emotional picker-upper, sending funny texts and emails every day. Yet another friend took responsibility for Lalee and was on call for whenever we needed carpooling or playdates.

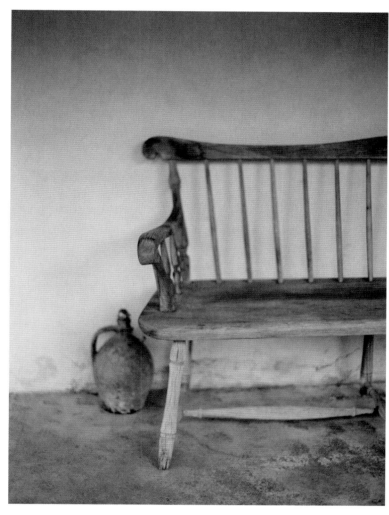

It was also up to me to identify who would *not* do what. For example, there were several people who couldn't, as Colonel Jessup said in *A Few Good Men,* "handle the truth." In other words, it freaked them out first that I (a healthy, athletic young woman with no family history) was diagnosed with breast cancer and then that I became as sick as I did. Being around this type of energy was not exactly advantageous to my treatment process; therefore, I distanced myself from these people.

On the other end of the spectrum, there were a few people who were "swoop and savers." These were the self-appointed treatment police who sought to stand guard and criticize each and every aspect of the treatment because their aunt's sister's cousin's doctor said, "Blah-blah-blah." In response, I found myself saying, "Please don't be my medical police. I need support, not your opinion and certainly not your criticism." The Silver Lining here was that prior to my diagnosis, I had never been able to say what I needed, and now I could.

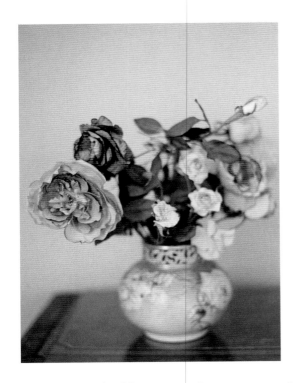

SEEKING SUPPORT

I was blessed to have an incredibly caring, thoughtful, and steadfast support system during my treatment. There are many people who are not so fortunate. Studies estimate that a quarter of cancer patients have little to no support. The resulting isolation can have a profoundly negative impact on treatment and outcomes, from missing appointments to missing meals.

In the absence of a system, it is imperative to find even a few people who can provide support. The Silver Lining is that there are lots of ways to seek and build a support network. Begin with a conversation with your doctor(s), either by phone or in person. An oncologist's ultimate goal is to fire you as a patient; therefore, she or he will do everything under the sun to ensure that your treatments work and that you get what you need in the process.

Many cancer centers and organizations have buddy systems that partner patients with volunteers who help with driving as well as food delivery and preparation. Online support networks are also a good lifeline option to stay connected and supported through these crazily difficult times. The American Psychosocial Oncology Society (APOS) has a toll-free help line (see the Resource Guide) to help cancer patients and caregivers obtain referrals to local counseling. Social workers, counselors, and support groups at either the cancer center or local organizations are another excellent way to help you get through. Please! Please! Please! Get the help that you need, the moment that you need it!

ACCOM(PAIN)MENT

Being with a loved one who has breast cancer is really hard. Though sitting beside the bed is not nearly the same as being in the bed, it is still rotten. My husband said that watching me being rolled into surgery for my double mastectomy was excruciating. One girlfriend called midway through chemo and told me that she had no idea what in the world to do (or not do) for me. It dawned on me that other people couldn't read my mind. *Shocker!*

Not only that, but during treatment, I had two dear girlfriends diagnosed with cancer, one of whom died. I found myself sitting (figuratively) by their beds, in a position of wanting to support, care for, inform, and guide them yet not knowing exactly how. Friends, I realized, also have feelings of confusion, sadness, frustration, and helplessness that patients do.

BEING WITH
(This is for you, friends & families!)

Be Present

Presence does not necessarily mean *in the flesh*. Presence means helping with child care. Dropping off food. Running errands. Being present means practicing random acts of kindness in the form of sending a note (via email or snail mail), forwarding a photo, suggesting a film, or proposing a book, poem, or quote.

I vividly remember that when I was sick, a friend gave me a loaf of banana bread, which is one of my all-time favorite treats. To my horror, our dog, Buzz, inhaled the whole thing without saving me even a morsel. I was devastated. This is not too strong of a word, considering that even the teeniest little thing can feel catastrophic when you have cancer. This same friend magically produced another loaf, which I then proceeded to inhale (and did *not* share with Buzz!). It was the little gestures of presence (or the grand ones, like producing two loaves of banana bread in a twenty-four-hour period) that were the Silver Linings in my life.

Another friend, Elizabeth Messina (whom you all know because she is responsible for all of the photographs in this book!) came over to visit shortly after surgery. As we were sitting on my couch, catching up, she looked at my chest and asked, "So, what do 'they' look like?" Since most of my dignity was gone at that point (because I took my shirt off for nearly every person I met), I said, "Do you want to see them?" She enthusiastically said, "Yeah!" So I pulled my shirt down and revealed my new "lady lumps." She responded by saying, "They're beautiful!"

> **LIFELINE**
>
> *When it comes to being a friend to someone with cancer, there are practical ways to Be.*

Now, Elizabeth's not one for hyperbole and I knew that she really meant it. She went on to suggest that she photograph me. She said, "I'm a professional photographer and I'm your girlfriend. I don't know what on earth else to do for you." The Silver Lining is that what started out as a gesture of friendship and love evolved into a working relationship that culminated in the book that you now hold in your hand.

Both examples just go to show that each person has a unique opportunity to be present, in her own way. What do you do well? Ask whether your skill set (talking? cooking? cleaning? photography? music?) would be helpful to the person who's sick. It's the little things that family and friends do that go a long way toward helping your loved one with breast cancer.

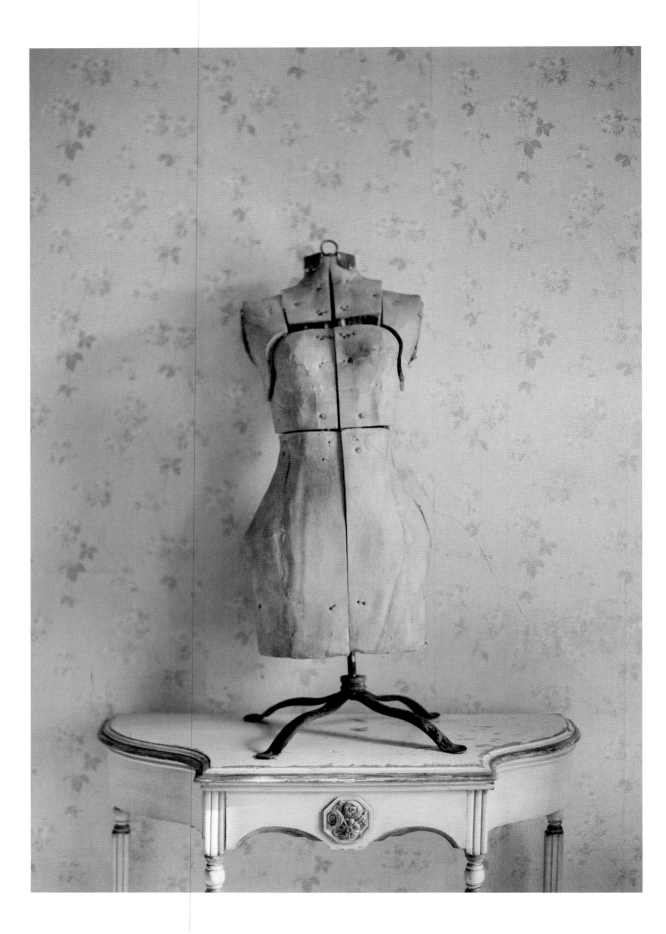

Be Inquisitive

Ask what would or would not be helpful. Just asking the question—being inquisitive—is incredibly sensitive, thoughtful, and generous. If your loved one is too sick to articulate her needs (which was often the case for me!), a Silver Lining would be to create a list of possible needs and ask her to simply check off what would be helpful to include, things such as:

- grocery shopping
- food preparation
- cleaning
- transportation
- weekly and monthly magazine drop-off
- babysitting
- pet sitting
- rake leaves, shovel snow, mow the grass

Also ask how she prefers to communicate. For example, talking on the phone made me nauseous, dizzy, and cranky. I told people that I preferred to communicate by email or text. I recognize that in the real world, it's not the most personal way to communicate, but when you're Puke Face, you do the best you can!

Be Patient

The last place I wanted to be was on Isolation Island. I love living in the world. I missed my friends and being a part of my extraordinary community, locally and globally.

When I was Puke Face after the second round of chemo and had to cancel plans (again!), a calm friend eloquently said, "We will all be here when you feel up for whatever you fancy." I can't tell you how much that sentiment meant to me. To know that those people near and dear would still be there on the other side of treatment was an incredible Silver Lining on the dark days.

Be Calm

Please hold all drama. Don't police the situation by criticizing doctors or making comparisons to your (or your second cousin's) cancer experience. There is already enough fuel in this fire. Whenever you can, keep things as light as possible. Now, it's not to suggest you avoid discussing challenging circumstances. Not at all. Just don't initiate them. Throughout this process, I intentionally surrounded myself with cool, calm, and collected people, which was a great Silver Lining.

Be a Good Listener

Sometimes I needed a good, unfiltered, tear-filled rant. It was hard to find someone who could listen, not because no one wanted to but because the subject matter was ridiculously hard. This was not your everyday moan-and-groan session. Rather, I needed to moan and groan about unfixable problems, at least in the short term. While listening, please do your best to devote your full, cell-phone-free attention. Please don't interrupt or say things like "I know how hard this is." Rather, nod your head and say, "I hear what you are saying" or "Tell me more." Use nonverbal actions like a relaxed posture or handholding to affirm a steadfast commitment to the (one-sided) conversation.

Be Honest & Communicative

Honest language has always been a moral imperative in my life. "Cancer" is a word that scares people. Most often this comes from personal experience. It's best to avoid comparing your experiences (or those of your brother's wife's friend) with the person who has cancer. Don't overshare. This is not a competition for whose circumstance was the worst. For example, rather than saying, "My aunt had the same kind of breast cancer you do and she was hospitalized three times before she died," you could say something like "I have an experience with cancer. Would you like to hear about the things that helped me and my family? If not, no worries."

In your communication, I highly recommend refraining from euphemisms. Use the proper terminology: breast cancer. One person, knowing that I had breast cancer, said to me that he heard that I had a "problem." *Uh-huh.* If our daughter, who was four and three-quarters when I was diagnosed, could say "breast cancer," then grown-ups can too!

Another communication suggestion (or rather, imperative) is don't ever, under any circumstances, use the term "only" in the same sentence with cancer treatment, for example, "You only have three more chemo [or radiation] treatments left!" When people said this, I knew that it came from a good and encouraging place, but it was like fingernails on a chalkboard.

Be Normal

Kvetch about the weather. Chitchat about flowers that are in bloom. Talk about the best (and worst!) dressed at the Oscars. Share the extraordinary things in your life. Witnessing a normal day and talking about normal things gave me a great deal of hope for what life would be like *after.*

Be Persistent

Many people told me that they "didn't want to bother" me while I was sick. While I appreciated the presumed sensitivity, there was nothing better than receiving a voice mail, email, or a card in my mailbox that said, "I'm thinking about you. You don't need to respond. Just know." I received these gestures every single day. They were not a bother at all. Rather, they were fueling, loving, and so deeply appreciated.

Don't Take Things Personally

My inability to communicate had absolutely nothing to do with what anyone did or didn't do. Rather, I was doing my very best to cope with the pain from surgery or the chemo coursing through my veins or the fatigue from radiation. Social graces go on hiatus during breast cancer. The things we take for granted in our polite society need to be forgiven because they are all but forgotten.

For example, I might make a plan at 9:00 a.m. to get together at 11:00 a.m., and at 10:30 a.m. I would cancel it because I literally couldn't make it. It was extraordinarily difficult to predict at any given time how I was going to feel. Within a ten-minute period, I could go from feeling moderately okay to being Puke Face. Canceling had only to do with self-preservation.

Additionally, I found that I asked the same question over and over and over again. Here was the kicker: I even knew that I asked the same question repeatedly, but I could not come up with the answer. Ever.

DEPARTURE

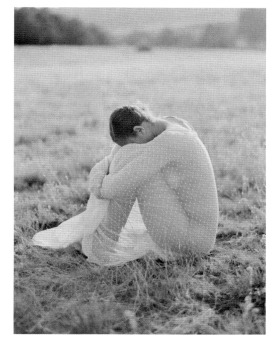

Leaving Isolation Island happened suddenly. One minute you're there, the next you're not. Departure is not without effort, a great deal of effort. It requires a commitment to leave combined with an enormous amount of mental and emotional determination. Departure also requires that you allow other people to support and care for you. Half of my challenge was just the release of control. Once I allowed myself to be cared for and supported, my burden was lightened and I was able to leave, which was a great and wonderful Silver Lining. ♥

No Man Is an Island

No man is an island,

Entire of itself,

Every man is a piece of the continent,

A part of the main.

If a clod be washed away by the sea,

Europe is the less.

As well as if a promontory were.

As well as if a manor of thy friend's

Or of thine own were:

Any man's death diminishes me,

Because I am involved in mankind,

And therefore never send to know for whom the bell tolls;

It tolls for thee.

—John Donne, from *Devotions upon Emergent Occasions, Meditation XVII*

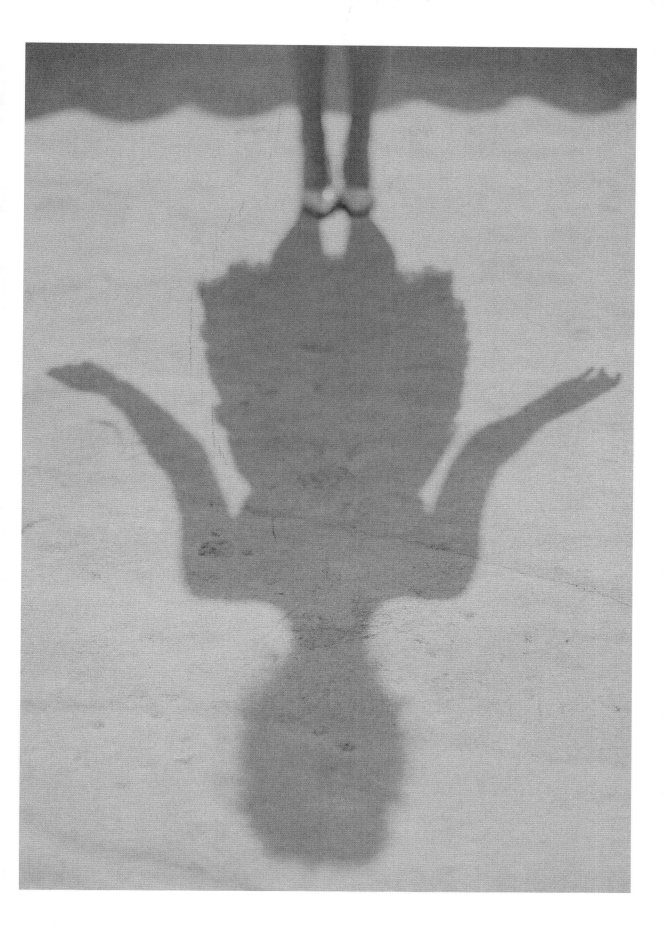

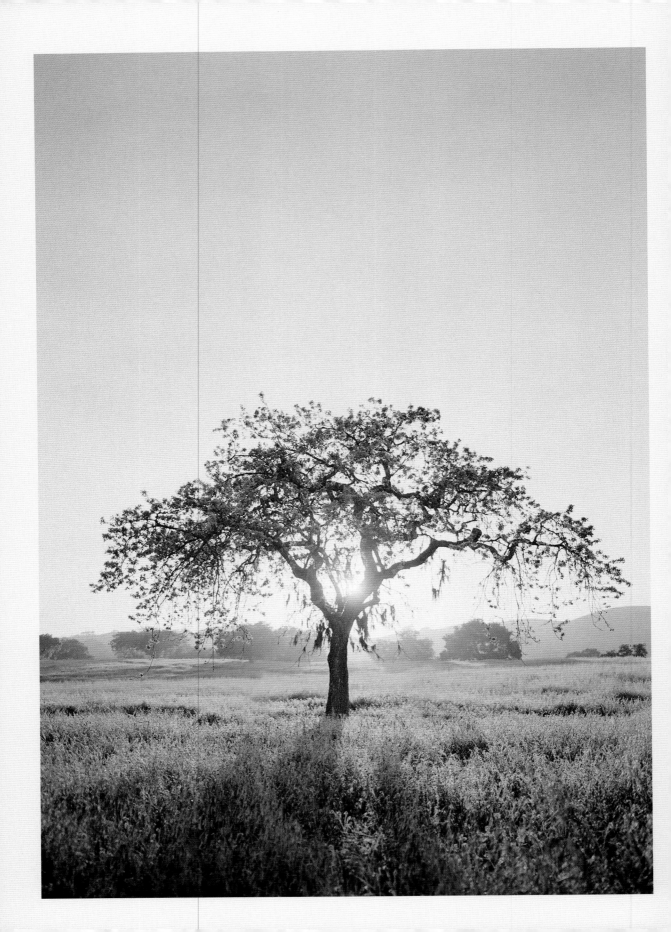

Support & Suggestions

NORMALIZE FEELINGS. The normalization of feelings goes a long, long way. Truly. Just the acknowledgment that wordlessness, attentional fatigue, and disorganization were my new normal helped relieve my anxiety immensely.

ARTICULATE FEELINGS. Talking (with both friends and professionals) about what was going on inside made me feel a little less loony tunes.

RELEASE OBLIGATIONS that bring you down. Focus on those people and activities that lift you up.

EXERCISE. Even the teeniest walk lifted my body, mind, and spirit.

ELIMINATE STRESS (as much as humanly possible!). Guided meditation and restorative yoga were two things that I did to help me rest, relax, and rejuvenate.

PLAN YOUR DAY IN ADVANCE. The structure will help you reorganize that which is disorganized.

SEEK SPIRITUAL SUPPORT through meditation, prayer, or rituals that bring you comfort. Guided meditation was immensely helpful to me.

USE GPS at all times!

FOCUS only on the things that are most important to you.

RELY ON YOUR SUPPORT SYSTEM. Allow family and friends to help. If you don't have a support system, you *can* create one.

BE OKAY WITH LEAVING THINGS UNDONE. This is a moment (or a few months) in time. There will be time to get things done later.

WRITE EVERYTHING DOWN IN ONE PLACE, ideally a journal. Please don't make the mistake that I did and use Post-it notes as reminders!

GET SOME FRESH AIR every single day.

CARRY A JOURNAL AROUND WITH YOU at all times. If need be, use Velcro to attach it to your body.

DO THINGS FOR OTHER PEOPLE. Send a birthday gift. Call a friend for no reason. Doing things for other people gets you out of your head.

WRITE DOWN AT LEAST THREE SILVER LININGS EACH DAY, from noticing the color of a flower to remembering your address to put into a GPS system.

CHAPTER VI

Radiation Cloud

*Understanding Radiation Treatment
from Simulation to Graduation*

Once my chemo was *done* and my PORT-A-CATH was *out* (very liberating, by the way), I had to mentally, emotionally, and physically prepare myself for radiation, the last leg of this long, pothole-filled road of treatment. The Silver Lining was that this was the *last* leg of my active treatment plan. Yippee-do!

After having a double mastectomy and chemotherapy, why do people have to have radiation? you ask. (Heaven knows *I* asked!)

When it comes to an overall treatment plan, one of my doctors encouraged me to think of breast cancer as a forest fire (a description that actually isn't too far off!), with each of the varied cells making up the flames. In eliminating a forest fire, there are firefighters, police, and search-and-rescue teams who have specific roles. Because one breast cancer cell is not like every other, the treatment modalities for breast cancer are multifaceted, just as they are in eliminating a forest fire. Surgery, chemotherapy, and radiation all play different roles:

- firefighters = surgery
- police = chemotherapy
- search-and-rescue = radiation

The difference between chemo and radiation is that chemo goes throughout your entire body, whereas radiation is targeted at the specific area where the tumor is/was. The goal of radiation is to either reduce the size of a tumor prior to other treatment or to decrease the risk that breast cancer will return where it began (in my case, the right breast). Because of my young age and the fact that I had lymphovascular invasion (the presence of one or more tumors in the lymphatic or vascular system), my treatment plan warranted a full-court press, including the search-and-rescue radiation team.

My radiation oncologist told me that if I chose not to have radiation, the risk that this breast cancer would come back (yes, I had to address the big *R* for recurrence) was 20 to 25 percent. Those are percentages that I was *not* willing to risk. Having the radiation decreased my risk for recurrence to 5 to 6 percent. My preference would be a *zero* percent possibility of recurrence; however, the lower numbers are oh so much better!

The people who are required to have radiation are usually those who have had a lumpectomy, a mastectomy with lymph node involvement (me!), or people with especially large tumors who aim to shrink the tumor prior to surgery. The timing and duration of a person's treatment depend on the type of cancer. Some people have radiation during chemo, though this is rare.

By the way, the words "depends" and "varies" can be very frustrating words to hear. While it would be easier to have a one-size-fits-all treatment program, the reality is that each treatment plan is unique and customized. So, as had been the case from the time of my diagnosis, I gave myself two perspectives from which to look at things: either the I-can't-believe-this-is-happening pity party or the positive, Silver Lining mind-set. I chose—and it was indeed a very active choice—the Silver Lining perspective.

Radiation works by using high-energy beams to kill cancer cells and destroy their ability to reproduce. Radiation changes the DNA of the cancer cells and

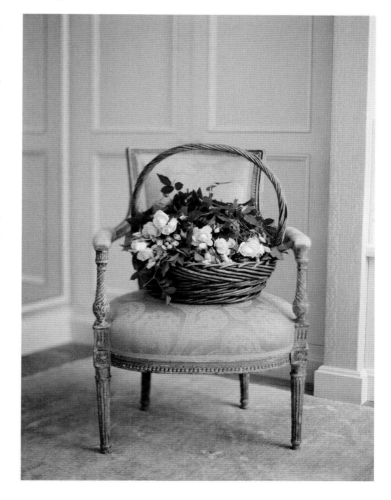

thereby prevents them from reproducing and spreading. The cancer cells die when they can no longer multiply, and the body naturally eliminates them. A Silver Lining of radiation is that healthy tissues are generally spared long-term effects of radiation because after treatment is over, they can repair the DNA changes, unlike the cancer cells.

There are two main types of radiation used in the treatment of breast cancer: internal and external. Also known as brachytherapy, internal radiation targets cancer cells by placing a source of radiation inside your body, either directly in or near a tumor. The material that emits radiation from inside the body is known as pellets, seeds, capsules, or ribbons. A catheter (a thin, flexible tube) is used to place the radiation in your body.

Brachytherapy is often pre-

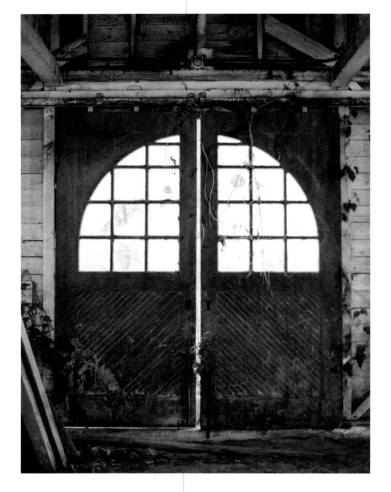

scribed for people who have early-stage disease, a lumpectomy, no lymph node involvement, and/or the tumor is no larger than 3 centimeters. Though this can vary, generally this therapy is prescribed for people who are at least forty-five years old. The Silver Linings of brachytherapy are that for the most part, healthy tissue is not irradiated, and generally there are fewer side effects than with external radiation.

The other type of radiation is called external beam (which is what I had). It uses high-energy beams to damage and destroy breast cancer cells. Though radiation damages healthy cells, the Silver Lining is that radiation negatively impacts cancer cells much more than healthy cells. In addition, normal tissues are shielded as much as possible while targeting the radiation at the cancer site.

My course of radiation was twenty-five sessions, which meant getting zapped at the outpatient cancer center Monday through Friday for five weeks. Twenty-five to thirty sessions are typical, though some people may have more, depending on the size and type of cancer. The reason for the extended, prolonged treatment is to deliver the necessary dose of radiation to destroy or kill the cancer cells and to lessen the damage to normal cells. The goal of scheduling weekends off is to promote healing of normal tissues.

The thing about radiation is that it takes time—days to weeks—before the cancer cells start dying, but the Silver Lining is that cancer cells continue to die for weeks and months after treatment ends. The delay in cell death makes a lot of sense, considering the fact that side effects can be cumulative and seem to hit (yes, you feel as if you have been hit) sometime during the third week of treatment. Some of these side effects include:

1. fatigue (a very familiar feeling)
2. dryness, irritation, and peeling of the skin at the treatment site (in my case, on the side of my right lady lump and under my arm)

3. increased pigmentation or darkening of skin within the treatment area (looks like a really weird tan)
4. temporary hair loss in the radiation field (I couldn't lose any more since I was still bald as an eagle when I started)
5. soreness or slight swelling of the treated breast and/or arm

The Silver Lining of these side effects is that they are nowhere near as bad as the side effects of chemo. Now, I'm not saying that the side effects aren't rotten (because they are!), but none of them left me lying on the floor of my bathroom because I couldn't leave my toilet.

There are three general steps in radiation treatment: consultation, planning and simulation, and treatment.

CONSULTATION

The first step in radiation treatment begins with a consultation with, and hiring of, yet another doctor. When you move from chemotherapy to radiation, your primary doctor is no longer a medical oncologist but a radiation oncologist (a cancer doctor who specializes in radiation). As is the case when you hire an oncologist, you never just hire one person. Rather, you hire a team of people. There are generally five members of a radiation team, including a radiation oncologist, a radiation physicist (the person responsible for making sure the radiation equipment works and who gives the prescribed dose of radiation), a radiation therapy technologist (the person you see every day who positions you for treatment), a radiation therapy nurse, and a dosimetrist (the person who designs a treatment plan that will deliver the prescribed radiation dose).

The HOTY (who at this point was still going strong as the Husband of the Year) and I went through the same process in hiring a radiation oncologist as we did with my other physicians. At each of the three interviews we had, we asked a whole host of questions to get a sense of the what, why, and how of my radiation experience.

I hired my radiation oncologist on the spot because during my initial consultation, after a physical exam and review of my ginormous chart, we discussed potential side effects. She said that because of my extraordinarily high sensitivity to

> **LIFELINE**
>
> *YOU hire your doctors. Treat every first meeting like an interview. Use your head & follow your intuition to find the right radiation oncologist.*

surgery and chemo, resulting in extraordinarily rotten side effects, she fully expected me to have all of the side effects of radiation and planned to stay all over me if not to prevent them, then to reduce the intensity of them. How's that for a Silver Lining?

PLANNING AND SIMULATION

This was the one appointment for which I was the least prepared. Oh, I wish I would have known what to expect! At this point, nine months into a miserable course of treatment, I was so doggone tired of appointments and thinking and interventions, that I (erroneously) assumed that a planning and simulation appointment would be no big deal. Boy, was I wrong. It wasn't devastating, but it did throw me for a loop. Had I taken the time and emotional energy to plan for what to expect, I know that it would have gone a lot more smoothly.

So, please learn from my mistakes. Here's the way to think about the planning and simulation appointment: it is the warm-up before the race. The reason for the simulation is that delivery of radiation has to be carefully and precisely planned. When I say precisely, I mean at the cellular level, which translates to a long, long appointment.

LIFELINE

Knowing what to expect before appointments is a Silver Lining because it demystifies and prepares you for the experience.

During this session, the treatments are simulated in order to determine specifically where the radiation will be delivered. The way to determine the treatment area is to use a CT simulator to determine exactly where the radiation will go. This is called a treatment field.

After changing into yet another unattractive hospital gown (with static cling in all the wrong places), I was placed on a long, hard CT scanner table with—here's the tough part—my arms extended in the most excruciating position above my head for an absurd amount of time. I felt like one of those helpless little calves in a rodeo, the ones who run out in the middle of the ring and have all of their hooves tied down so that they are immobilized.

After my first scan, I (erroneously, again!) thought: "Oh, that was easy. Where shall I have lunch?" *Nada*. I was in the room for just under three hours. The Silver Lining for you, dear readers, is that yet again I was an anomaly. It usually does not take nearly this long.

LIFELINE

Don't drink a lot before the appointment because there are few (if any!) opportunities for potty breaks.

And (I'm only telling you so that you can mentally prepare yourself, not to ruin your day!) you are in a cold exam room.

And you're alone. Why by yourself? you ask. Well, because the emissions from the X-ray and CT scanner are so toxic that no one else can be in the room. The technicians

LOUSY LYMPHEDEMA

After the tenth treatment, out of the clear blue sky, I noticed that I had the beginnings of lymphedema. My wrist was swollen and, while typing, I saw that I had an indentation on my wrist from where it was resting on the table. Plus my arm felt tight and it hurt.

I told my doctor about it immediately and, after confirming the diagnosis, she scheduled an appointment with a lymphedema specialist for the same day.

The lymphedema therapist gave me a "lymph massage" (unfortunately, it was all work and no relaxation). When I asked her how and why she thought that I developed it, she said that no one knows why a person gets lymphedema and went on to tell me that very little is really known about it.

What we do know, however, is that when lymph nodes from the underarm are removed during surgery, the flow of lymph to that side of the body changes. Consequently, the remaining lymph vessels have a harder time draining enough fluid from these areas, causing excess fluid to build up and result in swelling. The swelling is called lymphedema. "Clearly," the therapist said, "you are a person who gets everything." I was hoping that she would tell me something that I *didn't* already know.

At this point, I was already wearing a Spanx look-alike compression sleeve and glove on my arm (out of which the lymph nodes were taken) for air travel. This is standard operating procedure to prevent lymphedema. But now, as a result of my official lymphedema diagnosis, I was told that I had to wear the sleeve *and* glove all day, every day (when awake). I did get to take it off at night, however, which was a teeny Silver Lining. Additionally, I had to buy the next level up in compression-ness.

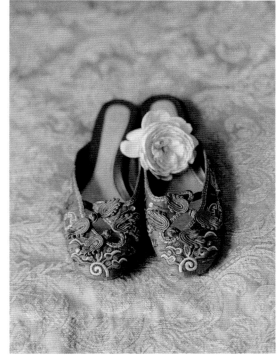

When asked "How does it feel?" I said, "It's extra tight." "Exactly how it should be," I was told. So now I had to wear an extraordinarily unattractive and uncomfortable appendage all day, every day. Fantastic. The manufacturer really should *not* put models on the outside of the box. They should advertise more accurately by saying, "Inside this box is a really unattractive sleeve that you have to wear. Sorry."

SIDE EFFECTS

FATIGUE At about two weeks into treatment—right on time—the freight train of fatigue took up residence in my body. One morning, I felt as if my arms and legs weighed 250 pounds—*each*. Whoaaaaa, Nelly.

While radiation is intended to destroy any stray cancer cells that weren't removed surgically or by chemo, it also bombards healthy cells on a daily basis. Therefore, the body requires *a lot* of energy for those healthy cells to heal from the damaging effects of radiation.

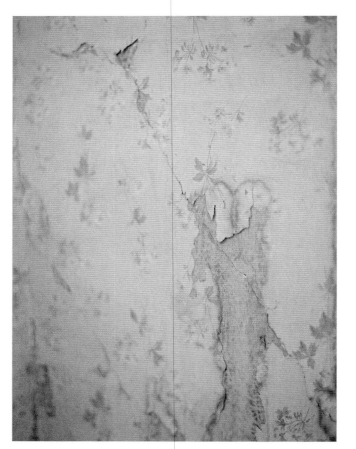

The best analogy that I can give is comparing it to spending a day at the beach—without the fun. Growing up, I remember spending endless days at the local pool (we didn't have beaches in the middle of Indiana, unless they were manufactured). I came home at the end of way too many days fried to a crisp. With my Irish skin, I tended to burn and then peel and then tan. It's so gross to think about now, but it's how I rolled in the early eighties.

At the end of those long, crispy days, I was so tired as a result of overexposure to the sun's rays. The radiation from a sunburn damages the DNA of the skin's cells, triggering these cells to die. The dead cells then trigger the release of inflammatory signals called cytokines that lead to redness, swelling, pain, and exhaustion. The same type of thing happens with direct radiation (without the sunscreen, I might add!).

Exhaustion was exacerbated by the fact that my body was expending overtime energy to repair the damaged cells. Plus, after surgery and chemo, I was already maxed out on stress and wiped out beyond words.

Despite the fact that I was so tired that I couldn't see straight, I was elated that I did *not* have to have any more crazy insomnia-inducing steroids. Additionally, I did *not* have any nausea from radiation. Those two *non*-side effects alone were enough to make me (emotionally) jump—no, leap!—for joy!

SKIN IRRITATION AND BURNING are very common side effects during radiation treatment. Once a week during my treatment period, I met with my radiation oncologist for a physical exam to monitor my skin. My doctor was meticulous about checking for the first sign of irritation and/or burn. At the slightest inkling of a change, she would vary my prescribed lotions and potions. She also encouraged me to wear soft shirts and tank tops with a built-in bra. My doctor also said to avoid anything with fragrance, deodorants, shaving, and sun.

These recommendations, I believe, made all the difference in the world. As a result, my skin held up during treatment. Though it was red, crispy, itchy, and sunburned, it was fully intact, with no blisters, holes, or gaping wounds. This was a gratitude-filled Silver Lining of radiation!

GRADUATION

On the last day of radiation, I received a graduation certificate. I have had the honor of earning quite a few graduation certificates in my life (because I love school). I can honestly say that this one meant as much as, if not more than, all of the others!

There was a great deal of emotion after my last radiation treatment. Walking out of the cancer center that day was one of the more freeing experiences of my life. I felt an array of emotions, including sadness, anxiety, confusion, and (obviously) joy.

The sadness stemmed from the fact that I knew I would miss seeing the kind people who had cared for me for such a long period of time. I felt anxiety: wondering whether the cancer was really gone and if and when I would start to feel like myself again. I felt confusion about what "myself" actually meant, as well as what the next chapter of my life would hold. I presume that there's really no need to explain why I felt joy.

At the end of treatment, I found myself looking so forward to serious downtime. I still can't get over how tired I was. Exhausted. Fatigued. Spent. Nothing quite seemed to capture the level of drain that I now felt. I often took two-hour naps twice a day and still went to bed by eight o'clock.

Radiation was the third of three legs of this breast cancer treatment stool. I am hopeful this stool will be a strong and solid foundation that will last for years and years (and years!) to come. ♥

THE SILVER LINING

There is no particular program
for coping emotionally with and **healing** the internal
wounds of breast cancer.

No regimen that can be prescribed with assurances that,
taken twice daily, everything will be **better.**

Treatment is a long, circuitous, meandering,
pot-holed process. However, I still continue to look for and
find **Silver Linings** every day.

Silver Linings do not negate catastrophic circumstances and
the feelings of sadness or anger that can follow.

What they do provide is
balance and **perspective.**

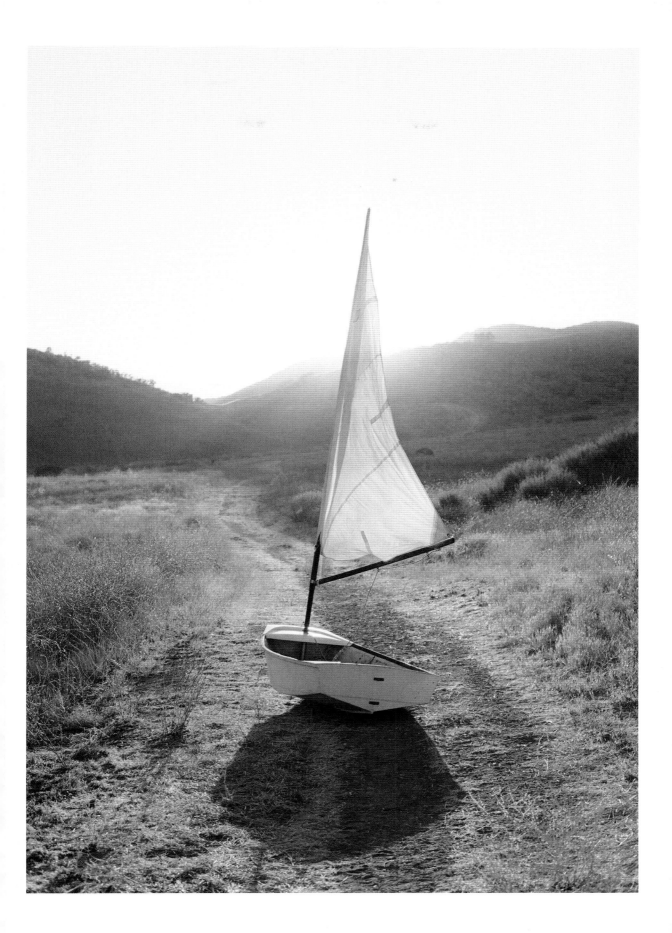

Support & Suggestions

- Be prepared for the length and discomfort of the planning/simulation day.

- Stretch before and after your planning session.

- Wear loose-fitting, comfortable cotton clothing that is easy to get on and off and won't irritate the skin. An oversize button-down shirt is a super option.

- Ask your radiation oncologist whether there is a choice between the two types of tattoos.

- Don't put *anything* (soap, lotion, etc.) on your skin before treatment.

- No topless sunbathing for one year. Sorry to be the bearer of bad news.

- No underarm shaving with a razor blade. This was not an issue for me because I still had no hair under there.

- Women who have larger breasts or who are heavier are more likely to have irritation or burning because of the extra skin folds for the radiation beam to pass through.

- Now is *not* the time to lose weight. Eating enough (but not too many!) calories and protein will help offset the side effects.

- Use birth control. If you are one of the lucky people who is still sexually active during treatment (yes, it is safe), be sure to use birth control because radiation is harmful to a fetus. And if you did manage to stay sexually active, please share your secret because I couldn't muster an inkling of interest, energy, or enthusiasm for any sexual contact. Hugging and an occasional smooch was as intimate as I could be.

- Ask for as many warm blankets as possible because the rooms are (usually) freezing. You can even put a warm blanket under you.

- Wear lots of sunscreen. All day (AFTER treatment). Every day. And reapply.

- Avoid antioxidants during treatment because antioxidants protect cells from damage. The whole goal of radiation is to damage cells. You can beef up on the antioxidants when it is time to heal.

- Follow your doctor's skin care instructions to a T.

- Communicate *any* skin changes, e.g., redness, swelling, or peeling, to your doctor and nurses immediately.

- Book the earliest appointment of the day. Even if you're not a morning person, it's worth it because early morning is the most efficient time in most radiology centers. If you can't book it early, please arrive on time to keep the system moving forward.

- Be prepared for the fact that fatigue can linger long after treatment ends. Please be patient with yourself and rest as much as possible.

Questions to Ask Your Radiation Oncologist

1. What is radiation therapy?
2. Do I need it? Why?
3. What are the advantages and disadvantages of radiation treatment?
4. How does radiation affect other treatment options?
5. What are the short- and long-term risks and side effects?
6. How can the side effects be treated?
7. Will it be best to have radiation before or after breast reconstruction?
8. What type of radiation will I have?
9. How many weeks will treatment last?
10. How will the radiation treatment be marked?
11. What is the likelihood of acquiring a secondary cancer as a result of radiation treatment?
12. Is localized radiation therapy an option?
13. Can I exercise during radiation treatment?
14. Can I work during treatment?
15. How shall I prepare for treatment?
16. What are your recommendations for skin care during radiation treatment?
17. How will effectiveness of radiation treatment be measured?
18. Will insurance cover the cost?

Ways to Help Manage Side Effects

EXERCISE. Though it is counterintuitive to exercise when you're so exhausted, my radiation oncologist told me that it is the number one way to combat the fatigue . . . and she was right! I walked and walked and walked every day after my treatment.

INCREASE PROTEIN CONSUMPTION. Frequently, I found myself craving salmon. It was a wee bit like pregnancy in that when I wanted something, I *had* to have it! I ate fish about three times a week and beans every day. If you eat meat, consume lean, antibiotic-and-hormone-free products.

SCHEDULE REST. I planned my day around rest periods. Frequently, I took a morning nap and an afternoon nap. I always ate dinner with the early birds and was usually in bed by eight o'clock. Yes, you are *that* tired.

COMMUNICATE. Be honest about how much you can take on in terms of work, social engagements, and family commitments. This is *not* the time to push through (as I am apt to do). When you are exhausted, rest is exactly what you need to do.

CHAPTER VII

Sustenance & Soulfulness

Nutritional & Complementary Therapies to Help with Treatment

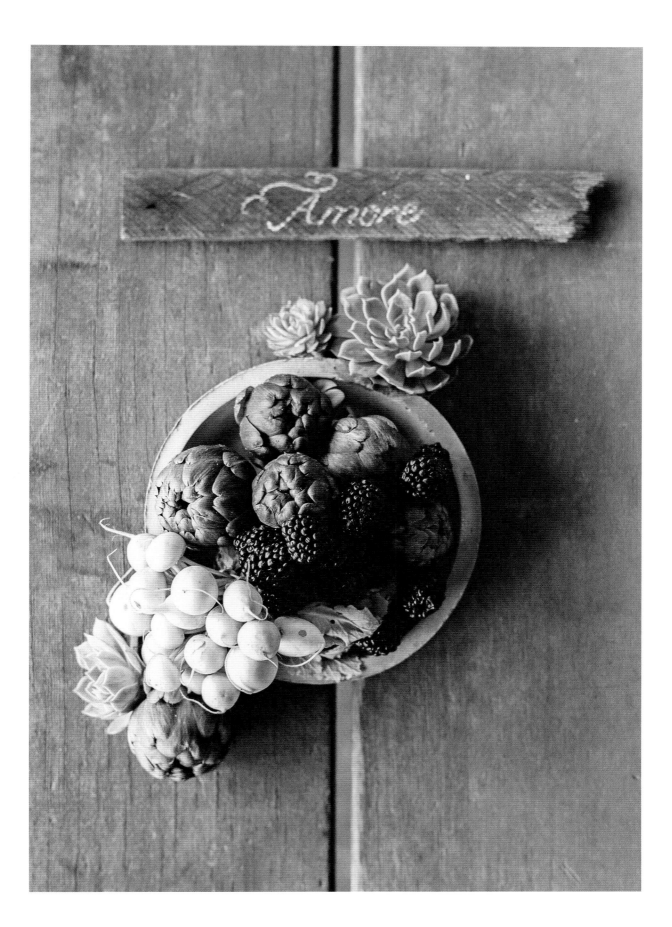

Sustenance and soulfulness were the Silver Linings that helped me manage pain, relieve nausea, buoy my spirit, and rest gently. When I was on Isolation Island, Sleepless in Santa Barbara, or nauseous at the bottom of the chemo barrel, it was nutrition, exercise, and complementary therapies that helped me endure the long and lumpy (pun intended) road of treatment.

Prior to my diagnosis, I had been pretty much vegan (though I ate wild-caught fish a couple of times a week and a random scoop of celebratory ice cream now and again). A healthy organic diet has been a priority for me for as long as I can remember. In fact, I happen to believe that it was my healthy lifestyle that prevented my breast cancer diagnosis from being much worse than it could have been.

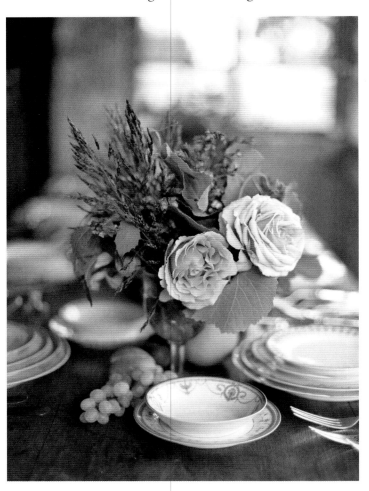

A nutritious diet during cancer treatment is humongously important because it helps manage side effects, enhance the immune system, rebuild tissues, and boost strength. Eating nutritiously is easier said than done because breast cancer and its various treatments can negatively affect appetite, food aromas, and tastes, resulting in an inability to eat enough of the right foods. Though this isn't the case for everyone, it sure was for me.

In the middle of chemo, when I was as sick as I could be, I found myself gravitating toward chocolate malts as the only source of calories that I could actually keep down. While I knew that I needed my vitamins and minerals in the form of fruit, veggies, protein, and fiber, my body was telling me otherwise, frequently in the form of "I want a chocolate malt *nooooooow* and nothing else will do!" The HOTY was only too happy to indulge my craving because he was so eager for me to consume calories—any calories.

There are several reasons why chocolate malts and other forms of sugar are not the optimum option for caloric sustenance during breast cancer treatment. To begin with, the sugar bomb that the chocolate malt delivered sent my body on a roller coaster of buzz and crash. As if my poor body weren't already contending with enough.

One day, while ravenously sucking down my chocolate malt and simultaneously reading *The What to Eat If You Have Cancer Cookbook* (yes, I felt schizophrenic), it occurred to me that I needed a real lifeline in the form of an oncology dietitian. I wish I had begun working with a dietitian as soon as I was diagnosed, but the Silver Lining is that engaging an oncology-specific registered dietitian is valuable at any point in the trajectory of treatment.

There are many different ways to find an oncology dietitian. First, ask your oncologist. Hopefully there is a dietician on staff at the cancer center where you are being treated. Another option is to consult the Academy of Nutrition and Dietetics for a referral. When you do so, be sure to specify an oncology dietitian. My doctor referred me to my dietitian and as it turned out, two of my friends had also seen her (and sung her praises!). Some insurance carriers cover the cost of dietitian services while others (unfortunately) don't. Be sure to ask your carrier as well as the practitioner.

Rachel Beller, MS, RD, the founder of Beller Nutritional Institute, literally saved my nutritional life. She was a magician who transformed my approach and ability to consume food during my treatment. Not only did she suggest unprocessed, whole foods that counteracted my nausea, vomiting, and constipation, but she recommended options that ultimately helped rebuild my physical strength and gave me a great deal of hope. What I appreciated most about her was that she told me what to eat, when to eat it, and where to shop. Considering her extensive experience, I trusted her implicitly. Her strategic direction took all thinking responsibility away from me, which quite honestly was a huge relief and special Silver Lining.

I had a tendency to undereat when I was sick,

> ### LIFELINE
> *Consult with an oncology dietitian from the time of diagnosis so that good nutrition can be a very regular part of your entire treatment plan. It will make all the difference in the world!*

> ### LIFELINE
> *A registered dietitian will be your guide to healthy eating when confronted with treatment side effects. Most cancer centers have one on staff who can help at no cost!*

which combined with my nausea and vomiting resulted in a great deal of weight loss. At one point getting on a scale made me burst into tears because I felt like I was literally wasting away. I challenge the pillow on my great-aunt's sofa that said, "You can't be too thin." I'm here to say that yes, a person can be too thin! Now, there are other people who, thanks to fluid retention, the onset of menopause, and/or increased appetite, gain weight during breast cancer treatment. Everyone is different. The key is, as Theodore Roosevelt said, doing the best you can with what you have where you are.

Some things that really made a difference for me included eating small, frequent meals, all day long. I would literally set my alarm to go off every two hours to remind myself to eat. If I had little to no appetite, I made sure that I ate nutrient-dense foods like avocados, grains, and nuts. I absolutely loved Newman's Own high-protein pretzels. I *still* carry those around with me for snacks.

LIFELINE

A big bang for the nutritional buck is drinking green juices & protein smoothies. The Silver Lining is that they are yummy!

I also prioritized eating fiber during treatment. It seemed as if from the moment that I took my first pain pill, I became constipated. This is a typical side effect from pain medicine, but for me the pain was much more debilitating than constipation. The Silver Lining is that there are lots of ways to counteract constipation, beginning with fiber consumption.

In addition to helping with digestive (plumbing) issues, fiber can be especially effective in ER+ breast cancer because it binds with estrogen (the hormone that helps cancer cells grow) to inhibit (or prevent!) tumor growth. How's that for a Silver Lining?

My preferred sources of fiber consumption were fruits and veggies (whenever I could eat them) and whole grains, especially oatmeal. A great boost of fiber can be found by adding ground flaxseeds to a salad, oatmeal, or smoothie. Speaking of smoothies, I made sure that I drank a fiber-filled smoothie every day that included oats, frozen

LIFELINE

During treatment, make fiber a top priority & best friend.

blueberries, frozen strawberries, spinach, kale, and almond milk. *Yummy.* Though I'm not a big fan of processed foods, I do like Gnu Foods Flavor & Fiber Bars. My favorite, the Cinnamon Raisin, has twelve grams of fiber per bar. That is pretty impressive! If you can't find them at your local grocery store, the Silver Lining is that they can be ordered online.

Dehydration tends to be part and parcel of breast cancer treatment; therefore, I drank purified water all day long. Right after my diagnosis we installed a (very reason-

touchy subject. Some people love supplements. Other people have an aversion to them. I personally fall somewhere in between. It is ideal to get all nutrients from eating real food; however, I know from my chocolate-malt-guzzling days that I was missing pretty much every vitamin and every mineral that my body needed.

The truth is that taking supplements during cancer treatment can be risky business. First of all, supplements are not regulated by the FDA, so you never really know exactly what you are consuming. Second, some supplements interfere with certain treatments. It would certainly be a big fat bummer to counteract the efficacy of chemo or radiation, not to mention the hard work that it took to endure them!

I had several friends who took supplements during their treatments and felt as if they benefited from them. The bottom line is that if taking supplements is important to you or if you feel like you simply can't get what you need from the food that you eat, I highly recommend talking with your oncologist and/or registered dietitian to see what could benefit you. They will be able to make suggestions based on your specific treatment plan.

Prior to my diagnosis, as a healthy eater and a nurse who took a nutrition class in nursing school, I (delusionally) thought that I had nutrition therapy covered. Ha! I couldn't have been more wrong! However, learning how to eat during cancer treatment is very doable. I promise. It takes patience, knowledge, and motivation. But with the right support, you can (and you will) get through it!

FINDING SILVER LININGS

Have you been wondering where this marked propensity toward finding Silver Linings came from? Well, it certainly wasn't because I am Miss Pollyanna!

The thing about Silver Linings is that they don't take away the (potential) side effects of breast cancer treatment, but they do provide balance and perspective. Pain and sadness are important and valuable feelings that need to be processed during and after any earth-shattering experience. The beauty of Silver Linings is that they don't take away the rain. Rather, they provide an umbrella.

Finding Silver Linings is a choice. Sometimes it is a really, really hard choice. There were excruciatingly difficult days when I had to turn over every boulder in my life to find one. For example, one day when I was in the bottomless pit of despair and found myself lying on my bathroom floor unable to move the six feet to my bed, I wondered, "Where is the Silver Lining now, Miss Silver Lining? You can't even get the six feet from this floor to your bed." At that moment—that precise moment—my eighty-seven-pound black Labrador came into the bathroom and curled up into a little ball right next to me. Two minutes later, the HOTY came in, sat down on the floor, and put my bald head on his lap. The Silver Lining was not that I could miraculously get to my bed. Rather, they gave me the love and support that I so desperately needed in that moment.

I have taken this incredibly valuable lesson of looking for Silver Linings into my post–breast cancer life. On frustrating days, when everything seems to go wrong, I look for the Silver Linings that I know are there.

EXERCISE

I have always been athletic, which is another reason why people were a little stunned when I was diagnosed. Hiking, running, and tennis are three forms of exercise that have always made my heart sing. Exercise boosts my mood, spirit, and body.

Between my first and second rounds of chemo, I went to (an insane) weeklong hiking boot camp that involved multiple hours of yoga and hiking a day as well as a "restricted" vegan diet. How and why (on earth!) did I do this? Well, it was a combination of things. First of all, I wanted to prove to myself that I *could* do it. Second, my soul needed it. Whenever I'm sad, grumpy, or confused, the best (and sometimes only) way for me to find joy, clarity, and enlightenment is to hike. Third, after having been sequestered for two months (postsurgery and after beginning chemo), I missed my girlfriends terribly.

During the first meeting with my oncologist—literally the first meeting—I told him about this trip and asked whether (a) the trip would be feasible and (b) if so, how. One of the reasons I hired him was because in response to my question, he said, "I'll do everything I can to make this trip happen." And he did.

There were an innumerable number of Silver Linings on the trip, beginning with the fact that I did it. This trip gave me so much hope for the future. During my long and dark days, I held on to the physical and emotional strength that I had during that week.

Spending this time with a group of strong, able-bodied women was incredibly inspiring and empowering. When I found myself in the bottomless pit of chemo despair, these women were my emotional, social, and mental buoys. They knew what I was capable of, and I believed them when they told me that I would get through the agony of treatment.

On this trip, I also reconnected to the spiritual part of my being. My spirituality comes from being outdoors and most of all from hiking. The air, the land, and the sea awaken in me all that is spiritual. At the top of one of the long, ascending trails

> ### LIFELINE
>
> *Exercise, even the slow stroll or restorative yoga, has the power to transform, not only physically but also emotionally & spiritually.*

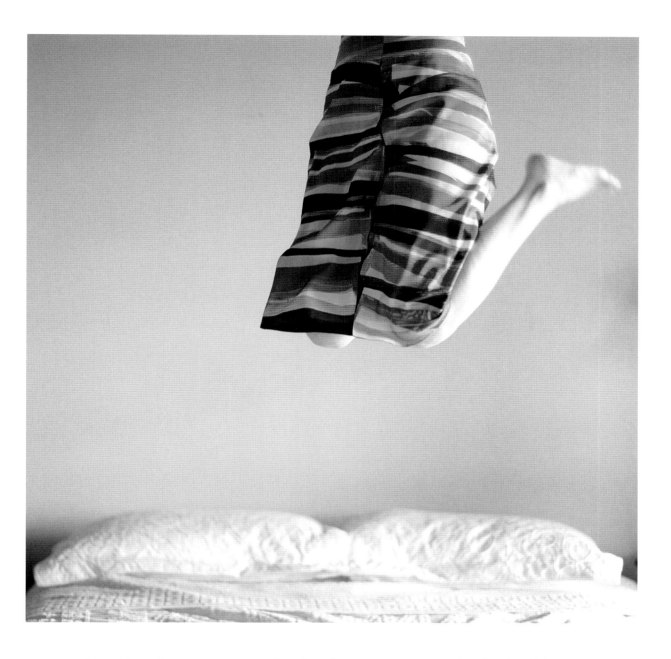

was a heart-shaped cactus. It was as if God said to me, "Honey, it is hard and will be harder, but underneath it all is love."

After that trip, though still a priority, exercise became a much more simple and gentle experience. Restorative yoga at the cancer center was my favorite form of exercise. I also took slow hikes, the Silver Lining of which was that I stopped to smell the flowers and look at the views. I enjoyed swimming laps in the pool (though not during radiation when my skin was sensitive) or riding a stationary bike. There were certainly days when I was too weak to do anything, but whenever I could move, I did.

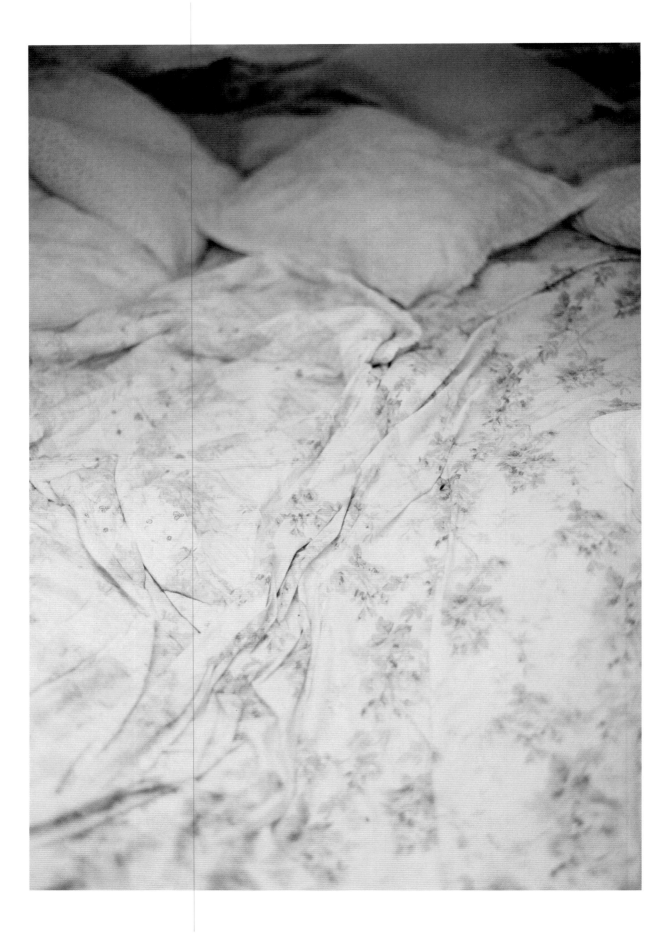

Zzzzzzz

Sleep, especially at night, was elusive when I was in treatment. Insomnia is common in people with cancer. Many of my friends told me it was one of the most frustrating side effects of their treatment because they felt like walking zombies.

It wasn't as if I didn't try to sleep during treatment. I actually tried every trick in the book to get to sleep, from pills to prayer, but nothing seemed to work. Getting sleep became a priority not only for me but also for my doctors for a number of reasons, the most important of which was because sleep reduces stress. When your body is sleep deprived, it goes into a state of stress. The body's functions are put on high alert, which causes an increase in blood pressure and a production of stress hormones, which in turn make it harder to sleep, resulting in a vicious, unproductive cycle. Those pesky stress hormones create an inflammatory environment, and here's the real pickle: cancer cells thrive in an inflammatory environment.

Sleep is also important because this is when the body tries to heal itself. The more rested a person is, the more likely she or he can tolerate the side effects of breast cancer treatment. Sleep also helps improve memory and mental processing. Additionally, because sleep and metabolism are controlled by the same sectors in the brain, getting enough sleep helps you to maintain a healthy weight.

During my treatment, when I couldn't manage nighttime sleep, I developed a power-napping prowess. When I was a little girl, I vividly remember my grandfather coming home at noon every day to eat lunch and then take a twenty-minute nap. He did this literally every single day. His routine and energy levels left a real impression on me and were a great motivation for me to try napping during treatment.

My best napping happened in the early afternoon, after lunch. My eating habits also contributed to my ability (or inability) to nap. For example, chocolate-malt-for-lunch days meddled with my ability to fall asleep. My naps were always better when I ate foods high in calcium and protein. I also found that napping beyond forty minutes made me feel groggy and undermined the reviving effects that a twenty- to thirty-minute nap provided.

I also darkened my nap zone (because darkness stimulates melatonin, the sleep-inducing hormone) by either closing the curtains or wearing an adorable eye mask that a girlfriend gave me (I think as a joke!) for my birthday. Additionally, because body temperature decreases during sleep, I always covered myself with a snuggly blanket.

I'll never forget the first period a few months

after treatment ended when I slept three nights in a row. I could hardly contain how happy I was. I did a happy dance every single morning. It was as if I were waking up for the first time in a long, long time. Though it takes patience and effort, a regular nighttime routine can come back after treatment. Pinky promise!

A COMPLEMENT

Complementary therapy was a huge Silver Lining in my treatment and helped with my incorrigible side effects. My doctors were very supportive of complementary therapy and in fact encouraged me to incorporate it into my treatment plan. My friends were instrumental in referring me to excellent, qualified practitioners for complementary therapy such as yoga, massage, and guided meditation.

Many people mistakenly think that complementary therapy is the same as alternative therapy. This is a definite no-no. Here is the difference: complementary therapy is used *with* or in addition to conventional treatment, whereas alternative treatment is used *in place of* conventional treatment.

Never for a single second did I even consider not having conventional treatment. As a nurse, I know firsthand its powerful lifesaving benefits.

However, complementary therapies also had a profound impact on my ability to cope with the anxiety, sadness, and physical side effects of my treatment. For example, acupuncture did wonders for my nausea. Guided meditation helped me sleep. Restorative yoga stretched my weary muscles. Massage relieved the stress and tension that I carried in my shoulders. Reflexology put me into a relaxed state. Not all of the therapies worked for me, but the Silver Lining was that many did!

FUR THERAPY

Between my double mastectomy surgery and starting chemo, we adopted a dog. I know it sounds crazy. Actually it *was* crazy. I mean, really, who in her right mind adopts a dog before starting chemotherapy? Oh, that's right, you're not really *in* your right mind when you're staring in the face of chemo.

Buzz, yes, I named him Buzz. After all, there were so many cancer-related connotations that went along with that name, beginning the day when my dear, beleaguered husband said, "Will you *puhhhhhlease* stop *buzzing* around?!"

Buzz is a five-year-old "career redirected" guide dog from Leader Dogs for the Blind. "Career redirected" is a wonderful way of saying that because of his certain disabilities (recurrent ear infections), Buzz was no longer able to stay in the leader dog program. He was and continues to be an incredible Silver Lining who came into our family when we needed him the most.

There is nothing better than four-legged love, and boy oh boy, did we get it in spades! He has a perpetual look in his eyes of joy, longing, and love. He gave me so much peace during treatment, especially on my darkest days. There was not a day that he was not glued to my hip. We would sit outside for hours together. Every once in a while he would gaze at me with a look that said, "I love you so much and will never leave you."

The goal of pet therapy (I prefer to call it fur therapy) is to improve the physi-

cal, social, emotional, and/or cognitive functioning of people of all ages. Studies actually show that friendly human-dog interaction releases oxytocin (sometimes referred to as the love hormone). Many kinds of animals are used in therapy, including dogs, cats, birds, dolphins, rabbits, lizards, llamas, and other small animals. In my clinical work, dogs tended to be the animal most often used (though I do know of a hospice that uses llamas!).

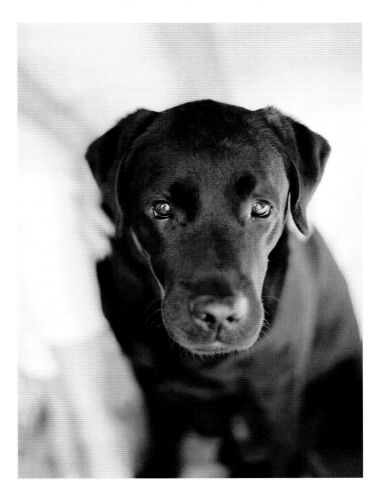

As a nurse, I witnessed the most astonishing transformations in patients during and after a pet visit. Many people showed an increased awareness, attention span, and interest in the world around them. I have vivid memories of how the presence of animals eased difficult conversations. Thanks to pet visits, I saw anxiety and stress melt away.

The extra special Silver Lining of fur therapy is that it provides magical feelings of unconditional love and support. Pets don't care how people look or what they say. They have no agenda and (unless eating!) are fully present. Heaven knows that of all the souls in the world, Buzz has seen me at my very worst. An animal's acceptance is nonjudgmental, forgiving, and uncomplicated by the psychological games people often play. They accept you the way you are, which is an incredible Silver Lining, especially when you look like something that the cat dragged in!

NO SHOULD-ING ON YOURSELF

How many times in the course of the day do you say "I should do this" or even "I should *really* do that"? Since I am of Irish Catholic descent, "should-ing" is part of my DNA. So much so, in fact, that I practically had to recite "I should" prior to my First Communion. My earliest memories include being told, "You should do [this or that]."

Needless to say, I am (let me correct that: I *was*) a big "should-er," day in and day out. I was always saying "I should go to this." "I should be here." "I should go there." "I should participate in that." "I should send the aforementioned." Blah. Blah. Blah. If you can't relate to what I just said, then *good for you*!

During treatment, a dear friend introduced me to this majorly fabulous concept of should-ing on oneself. Sounds gross, doesn't it? Well, when you think about it, the whole concept of should-ing *is* gross, not to mention bad for you.

Well, please allow me to encourage you from this day forward to stop should-ing on yourself! Now, let me be clear: there are certain things in the world that are not options—death, taxes, eating, breathing, and reading to your children. I also believe that being kind is a moral imperative that is nonnegotiable. Aside from these things, however, should-ing does not make for a happy life.

Think about it: do you ever really feel better after doing something you feel as though you "should've" done? I can honestly say that I haven't.

In some ways, I was a quick learner during treatment. During my time on Isolation Island, I was able to adopt this concept of not should-ing on myself rather readily. It's almost as if should-ing is seeing the glass half-empty, whereas *not* should-ing is seeing the glass half-full, which is the Silver Lined way to see things.

LAUGHTER AS MEDICINE

One of the greatest Silver Linings during my ordeal was the fact that I could laugh and often found humor in the utterly absurd. It was as if my sense of humor was literally on steroids (along with the rest of my body). From the time of my diagnosis through treatment and recovery, I continued to laugh. No matter how sick I was, humor made me feel better.

Laughing was magical because it eased my anxiety and helped balance the gloom and doom of my often omnipresent side effects and put them in perspective. Studies have shown that a good guffaw releases endorphins that result in feelings of euphoria and relaxation. I can't admit how many times I've seen the movie *Bridesmaids.* Perhaps it is because I can *so* relate to the bathroom scene. If you don't know what I'm talking about, go watch it. And laugh.

If insomnia hits in the middle of the night, I highly recommend going on YouTube and watching eight-month-old Micah laughing while ripping up his daddy's job rejection letter on "Baby Laughing Hysterically." It's been seen roughly 55 million times, so you know there's something special about it. It will be a fabulously hilarious Silver Lining of your sleepless night! In addition to watching videos, try as hard as you can to put yourself in a position to find humor, even if it means laughing at the absurdity of a situation.

CREATIVE OUTLETS

One of the Silver Linings of my being sidelined by my treatment was that it opened the time and space for me to think about and try creative outlets that I had never done before. For example, I started taking photographs. I took more photos of my backyard than I ever thought imaginable. There were several Silver Linings of taking photographs: (1) it was a beautiful distraction, (2) it expanded my mind and creativity, and (3) it enabled me to see the world differently.

I also started writing my blog, TheSilverPen.com. Though I had written clinically, I had never written personally. I found writing to be cathartic because it enabled me to release my deepest (and sometimes darkest) feelings. One component of my writing was my "Silver Lining Journal" in which I required myself to write down at least three Silver Linings of each day. This act provided some great balance and perspective on some dark days.

There are lots of other options. I know some people who found that knitting and needlepoint helped ease the numbness and tingling associated with chemo-induced neuropathy. Other friends turned to music to relieve stress and cultivate hopefulness and optimism. I have one friend who painted throughout her illness.

It's important to be aware of the potential for discovering talents and joy where you never knew they existed. Be patient with yourself, though. Go with what feels right and don't force yourself to do anything.

Of course, always remember, don't ever should on yourself. ♥

THE SILVER LINING

Sustenance and soulfulness

were the Silver Linings that helped me manage pain, relieve nausea, buoy my spirit, and rest gently. When I was on Isolation Island, Sleepless in Santa Barbara, or nauseous at the bottom of the chemo barrel, it was nutrition, exercise, and complementary therapies that were my Silver Linings to help me endure the long, pothole-filled road of treatment.

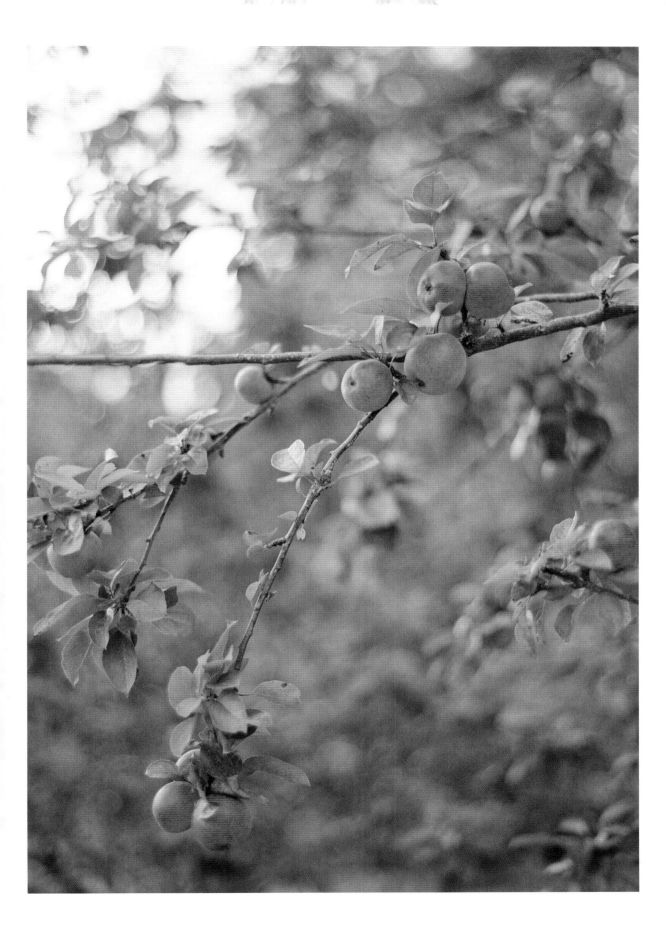

Support & Suggestions

- Choose to find Silver Linings on dark days. They come in small and big packages and will always appear when you look for them.

- Exercise has the potential to literally and figuratively move you, physically, mentally, emotionally, and spiritually.

- Prioritize getting sleep whenever and wherever you can. Partner with your health care team to use whatever means necessary to get sleep.

- Incorporate complementary therapies as a way to offset treatment side effects, relieve anxiety, and build physical and emotional strength. Be sure to keep detailed reports of what works and what doesn't.

- Welcome fur therapy into your life for a guaranteed pick-me-up.

- Stop should-ing on yourself—at all times.

- Laugh hard and often, even when things are absurd.

- Incorporate creativity as a way to reduce stress. Write. Read. Sing. Dance. Draw. Paint.

- Talk with your doctor before adding any supplements to your diet.

Suggestions for Eating During Treatment

- Eat small, frequent meals throughout the day.

- Eat even if you don't have an appetite.

- Keep your most favorite foods nearby at all times.

- Make healthy choices, such as whole grains, fruit, vegetables, and beans.

- Eat nutrient-dense foods like avocados or nuts whenever possible.

- Drink plenty of water (even if you throw it back up!).

- Make fiber your friend. Focus on fiber in the form of beans, vegetables, and fruit.

- Eliminate sugar and alcohol from your diet. Sorry, but you will thank me in the long run.

- Add protein to your diet to strengthen your immune system and help rebuild tissues.

- Make your own ginger ale by mixing three drops of ginger extract with sparkling water.

- Drink fiber-and-nutrient-packed smoothies.

- As much as possible, eat organically. Avoid processed, chemical-filled food.

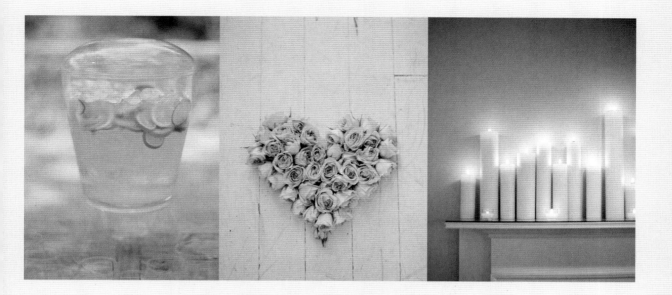

Ways to Maximize Sleep

- Give yourself a specific bedtime. Most adults need seven to nine hours of sleep every night, so take a look at your wake-up time and work backward to come up with a bedtime. Don't wait until you feel sleepy to think "Hey, maybe it's about time for bed." It's all too easy to keep yourself alert and busy way past the time that you should be asleep.

- Stay away from electronic devices for at least an hour before your bedtime. This includes television, but I happen to think that my phone, tablet, and computer are even more apt to make me feel artificially wide awake. I used to try to go through my emails one last time before bed, to get a jump on the morning, but I realized that this stimulating activity made it much harder to go to sleep.

- Don't drink caffeine for several hours before your bedtime, or even better, not at *all*! Even drinking it in the morning can make a big difference in nighttime sleep. I drink one cup of matcha green tea in the morning, and it not only produces Silver Lined health benefits but keeps me even-keeled for the day.

- Get ready before bed well ahead of time. I have been known to put on my jammies right after dinner. Not the sexiest look (well, sometimes I try), but getting ready for bed early helps guide me in the right direction.

- Create a bedtime ritual, and do it at the same time every night. Maybe you fix yourself a cup of herbal tea, maybe you read in bed, maybe you do an evening tidy-up. By doing the same thing every night, you will cue yourself to start heading to bed.

Ways to Incorporate Exercise

- Make the decision to adopt a physically active lifestyle by setting reasonable goals, for example: "Exercise fifteen minutes a day for the first week. Exercise twenty minutes a day for the second week."

- Be sure to write down your daily activities. It will make you feel good about yourself or motivate you to, *ahem,* pick it up a bit.

- Begin slowly but consistently. Start doing something—*anything*—for five minutes. This will establish a positive habit on which you can build. Sure enough, five minutes becomes ten minutes and ten minutes becomes fifteen and so on. Two suggestions: instead of taking an escalator or elevator, take the stairs; park at the far end of the grocery store parking lot and walk a little farther.

- Commit with a friend. By doing so you have not only accountability but also motivation! One of the things that I especially love about living in Santa Barbara is that when girlfriends want to catch up, they usually do so while hiking on the trails . . . talk about a win-win!

Complementary Therapies

ACUPUNCTURE: Traditional Chinese medical treatment involving the use of sharp, thin needles that are inserted into the skin at specific points on the body. It is believed to stimulate and alter energy imbalances and help heal and relieve pain and symptoms.

YOGA: Originated in ancient India, yoga is a system of exercises and postures designed to build mental control, physical strength, and spiritual peace using the body as the tool. Yoga is used to improve breathing, flexibility, concentration, and posture. It is also used to reduce stress and promote a feeling of being at one with the environment.

REFLEXOLOGY: A therapeutic method in which practitioners use their hands, thumbs, and fingers to apply controlled pressure to specific points on the feet, hands, and ears based on the premise that a map of zones exists on these parts of the body that correspond with other parts of the body. The electrical, chemical, magnetic, and nervous systems are stimulated with reflexology, which is said to boost circulation, increase energy, improve the immune system, and reduce anxiety, menopause symptoms, pain, and stress.

QIGONG: Means "cultivating energy or life force." Based upon Chinese martial arts, medicine, and philosophy, qigong is a practice of integrating awareness and aligning the breath with gentle rhythmic exercise composed of repeated movements known to strengthen and stretch the body. Qigong is said to build stamina, enhance the immune system, increase

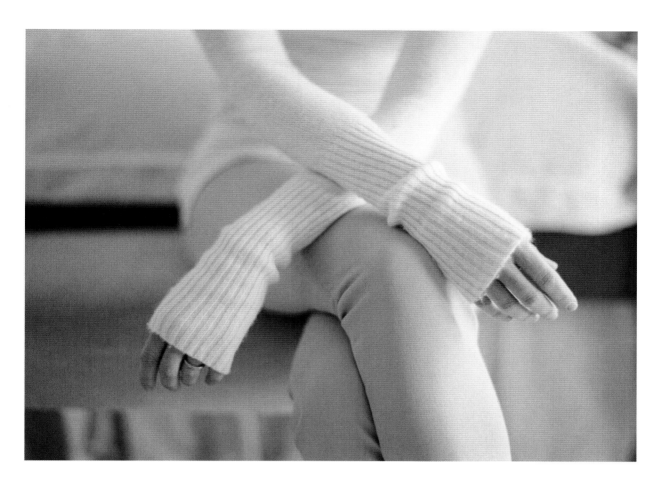

from my radiation oncologist was a sign of progress, success even. However, not having my daily treatments left me feeling static and alone.

The truth is that having treatment, doing something, felt easier than the uncertainty of waiting. Additionally, the end of treatment left me feeling as if I'd taken another detour back to Isolation Island. I felt abandoned and out of sync with the world.

REBUILDING

As I was grappling with the feelings of loss, isolation, and even confusion about what recovery was supposed to look and feel like, it occurred to me that having cancer is like being hit by a devastating hurricane or earthquake. After all, isn't having cancer one's own form of a natural disaster?

What do people do after their home has been destroyed by a natural disaster? They rebuild. The same thing happens after a cancer diagnosis. This process begins with thoughtful planning, including architectural and interior design with *you* as chief designer. During this period, I asked myself: What do I want my rebuilt life to look and feel like now?

It was a daunting yet exciting process, full of possibility. The Silver Lining of having my "home" flattened was that I could rebuild it any way that I wanted. I knew that it would take work, as any construction process does; however, it would be worth it because I could create the life that I wanted.

I harbored a great deal of naïveté (a lovely way of saying that I was delusional) about the recovery process. I presumed that after everything I had been through, there would be a lickety-splitness to recovering. I could not have been more wrong.

Like the home construction process, recovery takes a certain amount of time, effort, and patience. There is no set time frame. It will take as long as it needs to take. For me, it was a solid two years. Yet again, breast cancer demanded more patience than I thought possible.

NOW WHAT?

As soon as I started to feel more comfortable with the idea of being *done* with treatment and doctor appointments, the cancer center called to schedule an appointment with my oncologist. I wondered: Now what? More treatment? Remission? Testing? So, yet again, the HOTY and I made our way to the cancer center. Did I mention that he went to every single solitary appointment with me? How on *earth* did I get so incredibly lucky?

The "Now what?" question had two answers:

1. HORMONE THERAPY Tamoxifen is an antiestrogen (estrogen suppressor) medication that is a form of hormone therapy. Tamoxifen is given to women (like me) whose breast cancer is estrogen positive (ER+). It works by blocking estrogen receptors in breast tissue, which helps prevent cancer cells from growing. It is typically given after initial treatments (surgery, chemotherapy, radiation) have been completed to prevent the original breast cancer from returning. It comes in a pill form. I was scheduled to take it every day for the next five to ten years.

The common side effects of Tamoxifen include

- difficulty breast-feeding (so *not* an issue!)
- menopausal symptoms (e.g., hot flashes, vaginal dryness)
- irregular menstrual cycle
- osteoporosis (bone thinning)
- headache
- fatigue
- low (no!) libido

So, despite entering the period of recovery, I found myself embarking on yet another medication. As was my norm, I hoped for the best and prepared for the worst.

LIFELINE

Prepare for your first post-treatment appointment by writing down a list of questions to ask your doctor. It's also a good idea to ask a friend to join you at the appointment.

2. REGULAR CHECKUPS For the first year after treatment ended, I was scheduled to have blood work and checkups with my oncologist every three to six months. At my first post-treatment appointment, my doctor reminded me that no scans or additional cancer-determining tests. Only if I had any symptoms, such as pain without fluctuation or that worsened without any explanation, would additional tests such as a bone scan, blood tumor marker study, MRI, or CT scan be warranted. As a patient I wanted scans. I longed for tests. Scans and tests would, I felt, catch anything that was lurking. As a nurse, however, I know that testing doesn't catch a recurrence any earlier than does the identification of symptoms.

I would, however, resume annual gynecologic exams. The Silver Lining was that because I had a double mastectomy, I would no longer need mammograms, which meant that I had one—just one—mammogram for my entire life. Ha! The irony.

There is an inherent anxiety in post-treatment checkups. The first time I saw my oncologist after treatment ended brought on classic post-traumatic stress disorder symptoms, including a flashback to my first visit after my diagnosis, jumpiness, anxiety, difficulty concentrating, and trouble sleeping.

Before every oncology appointment, I am required to get my blood drawn. At the blood draw prior to my first post-treatment checkup appointment, I realized that my hands were shaking. The

LIFELINE

When you get your blood drawn, request a butterfly needle rather than the large ones that the phlebotomists typically use. The butterflies hurt way less! & yes, you can request what type of needle is used.

shaking made aiming for the vein a little, *ahem,* challenging! The Silver Lining was that I had a great phlebotomist.

What I came to realize is worrying really doesn't make a single bit of difference in the outcome of my doctor appointments. I made the conscious decision to see these appointments as opportunities to check in with my doctor. As a consequence, my pre-appointment shaking gradually subsided.

Another unanticipated side effect of treatment was the impact that it would have on my teeth. Teeth? you ask. Yes, I was just as surprised. At my first dental appointment after treatment ended, I was told that I had *three* cavities. These were the first cavities of my *life.* My dentist said, "It's not uncommon to see after chemotherapy treatment." Fan-flippin'-tastic.

MORE SURGERY

The next stop in rebuilding my after treatment was the surgical exchange of my expanders for semipermanent implants. As you may recall, when I had my double mastectomy and reconstruction, I elected to have the two-stage reconstruction, also known as tissue expander–to–implant reconstruction. Though the thought of two surgeries was a total bummer, the reality is that radiation can damage whatever is in its way. Therefore, my doctors and I decided that it would be better to have the radiation damage the (temporary) tissue expanders rather than the long-lasting implants. This meant leaving the original, post-mastectomy tissue expanders (which by this time felt like hard rocks under my skin and chest muscle) in place until the end of treatment.

Because radiated tissue goes through a recovery phase during which scar tissue tightens around the implanted expanders, my plastic surgeon recommended waiting about six months after the end of treatment before I'd have my next surgery to have the implants placed. Yet again, breast cancer commanded patience, but knowing that I was in the home stretch helped me immensely.

LIFELINE

Post-radiation scar tissue capsules commonly become tighter, resulting in discomfort, pain & annoyance.

THE NEW GIRLS IN TOWN

It took a great deal of research to decide whether to have saline or silicone implants. Implants are named according to what fills them. In other words, saline implants are filled with saline (sterile salt water), and silicone implants are filled with liquid silicone gel, which has the consistency of molasses. "Gummy bear" implants are another type of high-strength silicone implant.

Regardless of what breast implants are filled with, they all have a solid silicone shell. It is helpful to think of breast implants as being similar to balloons. A balloon may be filled with water, helium, or air, but it has the same pliable plastic outer layer regardless of what is placed inside.

There are many pros and cons to all types of implants. By all accounts, the best way to decide whether to have silicone or saline implants is to first decide which issues are most important to you. For example, the primary benefit of silicone implants is aesthetic: they most closely resemble natural breasts. In addition to being more expensive and requiring a longer scar, the primary downside of silicone implants is their potential to "silently" rupture, meaning they can break open and leak silicone into

your body. The most effective way to identify a rupture is by an MRI. The FDA recommends routine MRIs for women with silicone breast implants (but this is not consistent with all plastic surgeons' practices).

I decided to have saline implants because they are as safe as implants can be. The content of the saline implant is the same fluid that is injected into veins. In other words, if they leaked, my body would safely absorb the fluid (unlike silicone). According to my plastic surgeon, the decision was between "the total safety of saline-filled implants versus a (maybe) more natural feel of silicone gel." If I learned one thing during my year of treatment, it was that Murphy's Law was absolute with me: if something could go wrong, it would. At that point in my life, I was all about safety first and didn't want to take the chance of having a silent rupture resulting in an

> ### LIFELINE
> *Please talk in depth with your doctors about whether to have silicone or saline.*

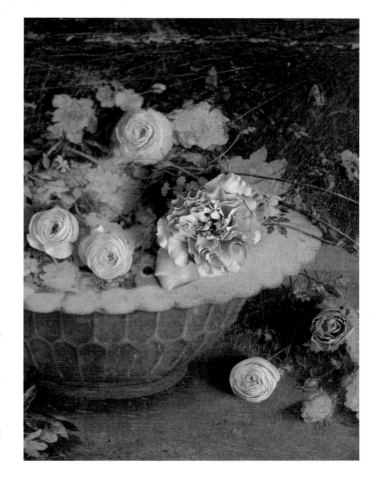

unnatural substance rummaging around in my body.

Surgery was a two-and-a-half-hour-long procedure under full anesthesia. I had a great deal of discomfort after surgery, which meant that I took a full-court press of pain medicine combined with copious amounts of anti-constipation drugs.

For three days after my surgery, my new "breasts" (it felt weird to call them that because they aren't *real* breasts, so from that point on I have referred to them as "the Girls") were wrapped up like mummies. The fourth day after surgery was the big "unveiling." The Silver Lining was that by the time of the reveal, my pain and plumbing were under control.

I was hoping that the unveiling experience would be a little like the scene in *Shakespeare in Love* when Will Shakespeare (played by Joseph Fiennes) unravels the tightly bound clothes of male-disguised Viola De Lesseps as Master Tom Kent (played by Gwyneth Paltrow). Too aspirational? Uh, *yeah,* just a tad.

Instead, my doctor said, "I need for you to recline in the chair."

"Why?" I asked.

"Well, because people have a tendency to hit the floor when I take off the bandages and move the new breast in the cavity." Really? *Really?*

While I didn't faint, I did see stars. *Holy moly,* did it ever *hurt.* Why? you ask. Well, because capsular contracture (scar tissue that builds around foreign materials inserted in the body) had already begun forming. So, my doctor demonstrated (an understatement!) the way to displace the implants to prevent firmness, and to create softer, more natural-looking breasts. (Side note: That last sentence reads so much more nicely than it actually played out!)

He assured me that I would be able to do this displacement every day. Not only would I be able to do it, but I needed to do it because stretching the scar tissue would keep the Girls soft; it would also break up small binding constrictions and create space to give the implants movement.

After the stars stopped dancing before my eyes, I was shocked by how *huge* the Girls were. At first it looked as if the wrong size implants were inserted, but what I realized was that the (big!) size was swelling related. It took several months for the swelling to go down. Despite the initial shock, bruising, and itching (another predictable post-op side effect), and the excessively unattractive surgical bra that I wore 24/7 for several weeks, I was so happy to be *done*.

Eventually, the Girls and I settled into a happy coexistence. I move my new breasts around in their pockets (aka "displacement") twice a day. In fact, it has become so automatic that sometimes I do the displacement while standing in line at the grocery store. Oh yes, I do. I can only imagine how weird that looks!

PHYSICAL TRANSFORMATION

One of the most important elements to add to the foundation of my new life was physical strength. Physical strength is something that has always been a priority for me. When I hike and run, I feel like I am more connected to the world around me. I am more grounded.

The morning after my double mastectomy and reconstruction surgery, the first thing I did was walk the hospital halls (even though I felt as if I had been an extra in *The Texas Chain Saw Massacre*). For the past year, my body had belonged to surgeons, oncologists, nurses, phlebotomists, insurers, and radiation therapists. My physical strength was zapped. I consciously decided that this period of recovery was my opportunity to return ownership of my body to myself.

One of the things that I did during the depths of treatment was to set a physical goal for after treatment. I decided to run a half marathon on my Cancerversary (the anniversary date of my diagnosis).

Running after breast cancer isn't physically easy. I found that running turned out to be even more challenging while recovering from cancer treatment. After treatment, in part because I was especially sick, my muscles had lost all tone and my lungs had lost capacity. However, my feet persistently clunked along, despite the aching of my knees and legs.

> ### LIFELINE
>
> *Setting a physical goal during recovery is a highly motivating aspiration that enables you to take back control of your body.*

After I'd withstood breast cancer and all of its treatments, the aches of running didn't hold nearly as much weight. There was absolutely no comparison to the pain and fatigue that accompany breast cancer. It is radically freeing and exhilarating to engage in physical endurance on my own terms rather than being subjected to the hardship of cancer. This sounds like se-*run*-dipity to me!

There are many Silver Linings of running (and physical exercise in general). It was really (really!) good for my post-treatment attitude, because it got me off the roller coaster in my head. Running, hiking, and playing tennis helped me relish what my

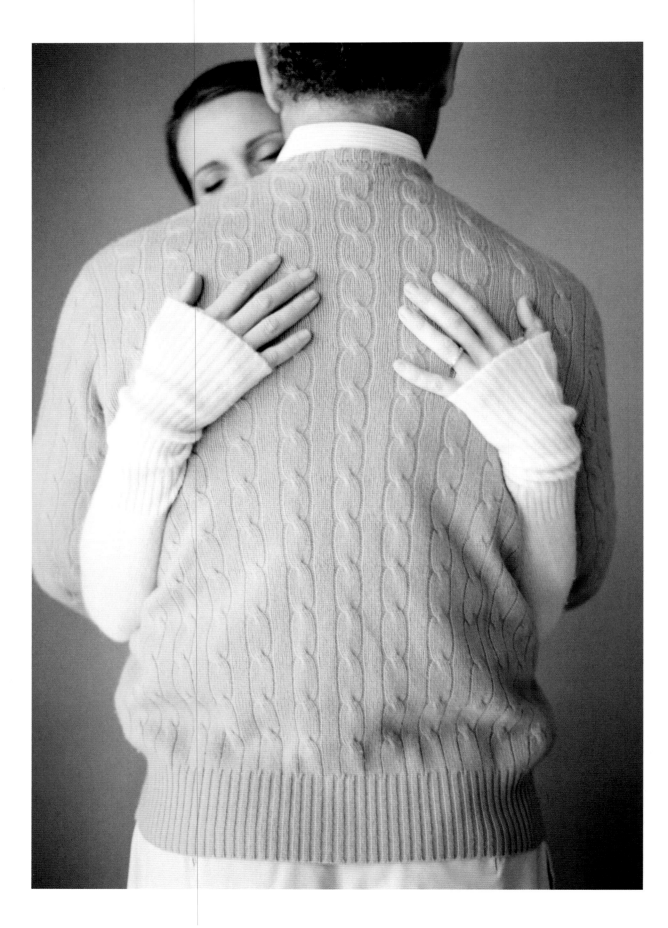

body could do now and in the future. They also reminded me of what I was able to withstand during treatment. I am now so much more grateful for all that my body and mind can do, especially when they team up and work together!

I finished the half marathon and cried tears of joy and relief as I crossed the finish line and fell into the HOTY's arms. The added Silver Lining is that the date of my diagnosis would forever be remembered also as the date (a year later) that I ran 13.1 miles!

RELATIONSHIP RECOVERY

In addition to the external building process, there was also interior redesign work that needed to happen during this recovery period. At the beginning of the book, I told you that cancer doesn't just happen to you; it also happens to your family, your friends, and your community. Well, guess who else has to recover?

Shortly after I finished radiation, the HOTY came into my home office with a stack of files and papers and said, "Here. I'm done." My first thought was, "Huh? What do you mean 'done'? I'm not *done*. My brain doesn't work. I'm exhausted. I'm trying to figure out what on earth happened to the last year of my life."

Fortunately, by this point my frontal lobe (the part of the brain responsible for controlling emotions) had begun working again, which enabled me to think twice before responding. Instead of an angry, sarcastic remark, I responded with "Okay, honey. Let me take a look at what you have there." The second he left my office I burst into tears. Then it occurred to me that I was not the only one who had suffered.

I knew it was hard for the HOTY during treatment. Never in my personal or professional life had I ever seen a more kind, sensitive, or generous partner. When I started to think about him, really reflect on his experience, I realized that he also went through hell. Granted, it was a different kind of hell, but it was still hell. After a year of holding down the household, being Mommy and Daddy to Lalee, managing our insurance and bills, schlepping my sick and sorry self to and from a gazillion breast cancer appointments, he was indeed done. I knew it and wanted so much to help him.

> ### LIFELINE
>
> *Be understanding of what family members have gone through. Relationships also need to recover from breast cancer treatment. Seeking personal & professional guidance is a productive & effective way to help you manage the roller coaster of recovery.*

The pickle was that I felt ill equipped to be his support when I was still in such a fragile state, still reeling with fatigue, chemo brain, and 'roid rage. I decided that I needed some professional guidance to help me find the proper balance in our marriage after the diagnosis and treatment. I also reached out to LiFT and another friend who had recently gone through the recovery process.

My therapist and my friends informed me that my feelings of inadequacy were as normal as his feelings of frustration. Talk about being between a rock and a hard place. They all gently suggested (reminded me, actually) that communication is the first step in the recovery of a relationship. So, the HOTY and I started talking. It was hard at first, but the more open and communicative we were, the better our relationship became.

Though Lalee weathered my treatment as well as she could have, after I finished treatment, she became a stage five clinger. She was also done with breast cancer. Lalee was acutely aware that treatment was over and needed me to be fully present, from making breakfast in the morning to reading books to her before bed. She was eager and excited for me to go to the park with her and play. There was no greater Silver Lining than to be able to do so with her.

During recovery, Lalee and I continued to talk about breast cancer. Because I had drilled into her head that cancer is not contagious, that she did nothing to cause it, and that she would be cared for when I was sick, those issues didn't arise again. Our conversations revolved around what life would now be like. She asked:

"When will your hair grow back?"

"It takes time, but hopefully by the time you go back to school in the fall, I will have my hair back," I said.

"When will you have more energy?"

"Soon, I hope. I have a little more energy every day," I said.

"Why does it take so long to feel better?"

"The medicines that I took were very, very strong. It killed the cancer cells, but it also killed many of my healthy cells. It takes a lot of time to make more cells. But the Silver Lining is that the cells do come back."

I was happy, thrilled actually, that Lalee continued to share what was on her mind and in her heart. Not all children are this communicative; however, gentle and persistent encouragement to ask questions and talk about what they are thinking and feeling is not only helpful in opening the doors of dialogue, but it also affirms that you are there for them whenever and wherever they need to express themselves.

Relationship recovery began with my family, my core. During my (really, *our*) recovery process, I put my full faith and trust in the belief that if I could be emotionally, mentally, and physically present for Lalee and the HOTY, then we would *all* recover. This was the ultimate Silver Lining.

COMING-OUT PARTY

Having been sequestered on Isolation Island for a lot of the past year, I was eager and excited to reacquaint myself with friends whom I hadn't seen in, well, about a year. I erroneously thought that seeing everyone all at one time at a big community event would be a fantabulous way to catch up and put myself back in the mainstream. Breast cancer laughed at me—*again*.

About six months into recovery, we were invited to a ginormous, fancy-schmancy black-tie event. The HOTY is especially handsome in a tuxedo and I love wearing a long gown, so I was excited to go. Socially, I felt ready to reconnect and reengage.

At the party, a friend referred to my attendance as my coming-out party (because I hadn't seen most of these people since before my diagnosis). Prior to the party, I spent a lot more time than usual focusing on my personal appearance; subconsciously, I knew that it was indeed my coming-out party.

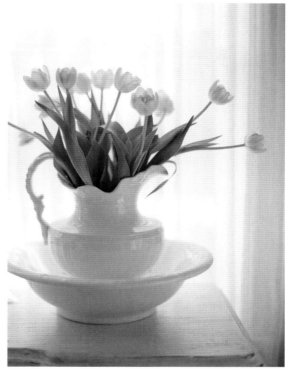

Seeing people for the first time after having been sick is a unique experience. With their heads turned sideways, people ask, "How *arrrrrrrrrre* you?" I consistently felt compelled to put their worries at ease and generally put on my biggest smile and say, "Great!" because the truth of the matter is that is what people want to hear. People didn't want to know that I was totally wiped out and that there were residual side effects to my year with breast cancer. People wanted to hear and believe that life was back to normal, as if nothing had happened.

One way in which breast cancer changed me is that I am less comfortable grinning and gripping in crowds. I'm no longer a schmoozer (not that I was really a full schmoozer before, but I could definitely work a room). Rather, I prefer being in small groups of people. Additionally, I no longer "should" on myself. For example, before dinner, when people were mingling (read: schmoozing!), I felt like sitting down. I was happy as a clam, actually, just sitting at a table, by myself. What a Silver Lining to eliminate any and all feelings of obligation.

I did the best that I could and made it through the party, though I left early, during dessert, because I was so physically and emotionally exhausted. I learned a valuable lesson from that party: my head, heart, and body were still out of sync. My socially starved self wanted so much to reengage with friends, but emotionally and physically, I wasn't ready to do so on such a large scale. Therefore, I decided that I needed to rein things in a bit and reconnect on a smaller scale, with a few friends at a time rather than in a large group. The Silver Lining of this approach is that you are able to have deeper, more meaningful conversations at a feasible pace.

MIND GAMES

Once my muscles were reinvigorated and my relationships rebooted, I knew that it was time to up the ante on my persistently pervasive chemo brain. My brain fog and forgetfulness seemingly started the moment that I heard the words, "You have breast cancer" and persisted, relentlessly. Some days it royally ticked me off. Other days it panicked me (especially when I was told that chemo brain can last for years)!

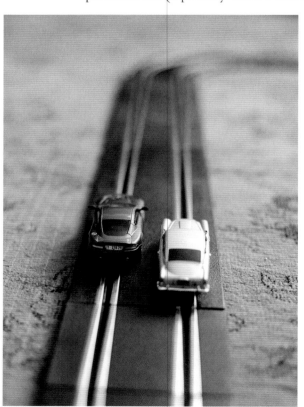

In my effort to take an active role in my own wellness, my goal was and continues to be to do everything I can possibly do to counteract my brain drain. Research consistently points to mental stimulation and brain training as a way to develop new nerve pathways to maintain healthy brain function throughout life.

My mind games included a multitude of things. Thanks to the lousy lymphedema in my right arm (where I had fifteen lymph nodes removed), I switched from playing tennis with my right hand to my left. It takes so much more focus and attention to play this way and I love it. I also started taking conversational French lessons with a girlfriend. I began branching out in the kitchen and experimenting with new recipes. I also started doing puzzles and brainteasers. I'm usually not good at these types of exercises. And truth be told, they often frustrate the bejeezus out of me. However, in my quest to eliminate chemo brain, it was worth it.

SURVIVOR GUILT

Though at the time of my diagnosis, I was shocked, I never actually wondered *why* I was diagnosed with cancer. I have frequently been asked, "Why on earth would *you,* a young, healthy, happy person with no family history, get breast cancer?" Even when *other* people wondered, I never did. I guess I figured that why wasn't the point. I had cancer. I had to deal with it. I had to look and move forward.

During recovery, I had two friends die of cancer. Both were young, healthy, and happy people with no family history. My question (to which there is absolutely no answer) is: "Why did I get what I got (a rotten but treatable cancer) and they got what they got (a life-limiting form of cancer)?"

I thought about this every single day. Sometimes this thought made me feel sad. Sometimes it made me feel scared. Sometimes it made me feel guilty. Yet again, clinical experience informed my personal one. I knew that I was experiencing a version of survivor guilt, a common experience for those who have survived a major disaster. And if a cancer diagnosis isn't a disaster, I don't know what is!

Here are three things I know for sure:

1. Anyone who has had a cancer diagnosis is forever changed.
2. Though not everyone experiences guilt, for those who do, it is important to know that these feelings are a normal part of this experience.
3. Unfortunately, survivor guilt brings with it a host of issues that can cause depression, anger, and self-blame, which may even compromise health. *Ugh.* Getting professional help to get you through this period will be your Silver Lining.

Now, please don't get me wrong. I was thrilled to be recovering. I don't know what's in my future. None of us does. But through this ordeal, I have faced fears, challenges, and heartbreak. I know that I have also learned lessons I couldn't have learned any other way.

What I now know firsthand is that life is a precious gift. After my years as a hospice nurse actually, I already knew that. I guess it's just been reiterated—in a *big way.* I have been given the opportunity to recommit myself to this belief, which is a Silver Lining in and of itself. My time to go will come around eventually, but for now, I told myself, it is my time to live.

DRUG HOLIDAY

As was the case with each and every one of my treatments, I had virtually every single side effect of Tamoxifen, including bone pain, headaches, coughing, hot flashes, muscle pain, nausea, zippo libido, fatigue, and vaginal dryness. So, after six months on Tamoxifen, I made a pretty radical decision: I decided (with the support of my physicians) to take a "drug holiday."

My biggest, most troublesome issues were and continue to be the hot flashes and fatigue. I had four to five *big,* drench-filled, disabling hot flashes almost every *hour,* day and night. The hot flashes resulted in an inability to think, sleep, or function with any remote sense of efficacy. And since beginning Tamoxifen, all day, every day, I felt utterly exhausted, yet unable to sleep. So, basically, I hadn't slept in a year and a half, and for the record, I'm a *disaster* without sleep.

After six months on the drug, I had a bleary-eyed conversation with my oncologist about whether I really needed to take Tamoxifen. From the time of my diagnosis, I'd never been one to sit on the sidelines and do as told.

In response to my question, he suggested that we use Adjuvant! Online to assess whether Tamoxifen was right for me. According to the website, "The purpose of Adjuvant! is to help [cancer] health professionals and patients with early cancer discuss the risks and benefits of getting additional therapy (adjuvant therapy: usually chemotherapy, hormone therapy, or both) after surgery." These estimates (including the potential for recurrence and mortality) are based on information entered about individual patients and their tumors (for example, patient age, tumor size, nodal involvement, histologic grade, etc.). These estimates are then provided on printed sheets in simple graph and text formats to be used in consultations.

So we put in every bit of my data and Adjuvant! estimated that the likelihood that Tamoxifen would prevent mortality or relapse within the next five years was 2 percent. Seriously? That's *it?* I thought. It was quite stunning and revealing.

One might argue, "But isn't 2 percent worth it?" My answer was no, not really (that's how debilitated I felt). My doctor said that sleep was more of a priority for me at the time. He told me that prolonged sleep deprivation has the potential to contribute to a cancer recurrence (he didn't give me a percentage on that). He then suggested that a "drug holiday" might be worth trying to see whether it was the Tamoxifen that was the culprit for all of the side effects or whether it was because of lingering chemo effects.

After getting a corroborating consulting opinion (*always* a great idea when making a big decision), the HOTY and I had a long discussion about whether this was the

LIFELINE

Be an active participant in your care. Ask the tough questions.

right course of action for me. We both agreed that the holiday and my quality of life after all I had been through was worth the 2 percent higher risk.

After agreeing to this holiday, my doctor reassured me in my decision by saying, "If you have a recurrence, it will *not* be because of this drug holiday." His reassurance was a Silver Lining to a difficult decision.

This is in no way a recommendation for you to take a drug holiday. Rather, my situation further reiterates the need to have a true partnership with your physician(s). Having these discussions about your health is imperative. None of this is easy. It never has been and never will be. However, the Silver Lining is that there *are* options!

GET YOUR SEXY BACK

One of the most challenging side effects of my breast cancer treatment was the impact on my sexuality. It was certainly understandable to lose my lust(er) during treatment. Certainly the physical pain of having my breasts lopped off validated the loss of any

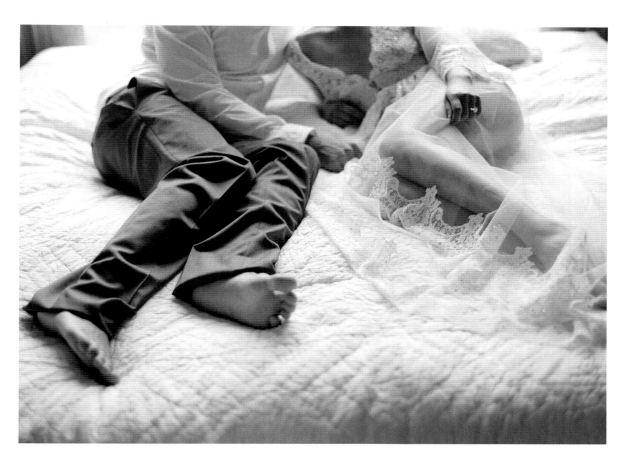

desire to hug. And certainly the chemotherapy-induced menopause resulting in vaginal dryness, hot flashes, sleep deprivation, and mood swings, not to mention looking like a prepubescent girl thanks to the hair loss, dampened any hankering for hanky-panky. And certainly the freight train of fatigue that came with radiation eliminated any proclivity toward frolicking.

During recovery, however, I hoped beyond all hope that my interest in and enjoyment of sex would magically reappear. Unfortunately, that's not how recovery works. Not only was sex not a top priority, it hurt like holy hell, which resulted in a double whammy.

Even though I knew that this was a biochemical situation, I felt emotionally rotten. Prior to my diagnosis, the HOTY and I had a very healthy sexual relationship. And now: nothing. I felt as if I was in the Sahara of Sexuality.

To add insult to sexual injury, being on Tamoxifen meant that I would be in this estrogen deficit for up to ten years! Now, the Silver Lining is that the less estrogen in my body, the less food for any potential microscopic breast cancer cells circulating in my body. The other Silver Lining was that I'm not alone in the Sahara of Sexuality. Research confirms that sexual dysfunction is common after treatment and especially in women taking estrogen inhibitors.

So, what does it take to get your sexy back? The first thing that I did (and continue to do) was to communicate with the HOTY. Though talking doesn't exactly turn me on, it enables us both to fully express our feelings, and this goes a long way in our relationship.

Much in the same way that I've been proactive in getting my mind and my body reassembled, I took an active role in rekindling the love(making) machine. I started by making a conscious decision to prioritize my sexuality. I've done things like purchase beautiful silk lingerie that makes me feel very va-va-voom. The lack of lubrication is remedied by a number of products on the market, including Moist Again, Astroglide, and K-Y Liquid. I also talked with one of my doctors about my unfortunate detour to the Sahara. She encouraged me to bring some toys and massage lotions into our relationship, which resulted in a pretty significant awakening.

Though the process is slow going, it does happen. It really and truly does. The key is to be simultaneously proactive in the reintroduction of sexuality to your life and patient with yourself, knowing that you can indeed be a beautiful, sexual person again.

> **LIFELINE**
>
> *Honest & open communication with your partner is what will help you get through the Sahara of Sexuality.*

CANCER IS NOT A GIFT

About nine months into recovery, I chuckled to myself when I thought about all of the people who had said (in different iterations) to me, "Cancer is a gift. Look at what you are doing now. You would never have done this if you hadn't had cancer." Yes, people said this. When this would happen, my cheeks would instantly turn fifty shades of (not grey but) red. I'd do my polite smile and take a deep breath before saying, "*In. No. Way. Is. Cancer. A. Gift.*"

Breast cancer does not have any of the markings of a traditional gift. There is no ribbon. No card. No love. No fun. And it comes with lots and lots of strings attached.

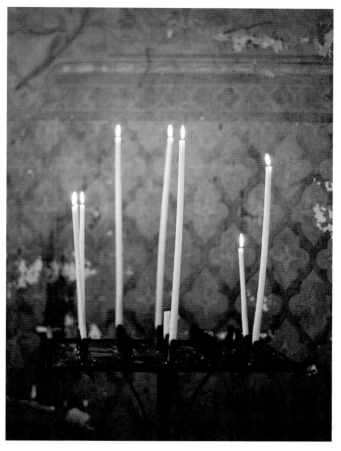

Cancer does, however, keep on giving. At a recent appointment, my oncologist and I discussed the realistic practicality of a prophylactic oophorectomy (preventing cancer recurrence by surgically removing my estrogen-producing ovaries), resulting in yet another tributary on this long, potholed road that is breast cancer.

Now, as you know, I have found an immense number of Silver Linings during my experience with breast cancer. Maybe this is what people really mean when they use the word "gift" (?!). I don't know and don't care to delve into a discussion (argument?) with anyone who thinks that cancer is a gift. I just can't go there and am not going to should myself on the topic.

What I know for sure is that Silver Linings have always provided balance and perspective for me. They have not ever taken away the pain, nausea, sadness, or isolation that came with cancer. The Silver Linings that I experienced during my cancer diagnosis, treatment, and recovery helped me get through each and every day. I have a tremendous amount of gratitude for the Silver Linings, but you'll never, ever, not in a million years, hear me refer to cancer as a gift.

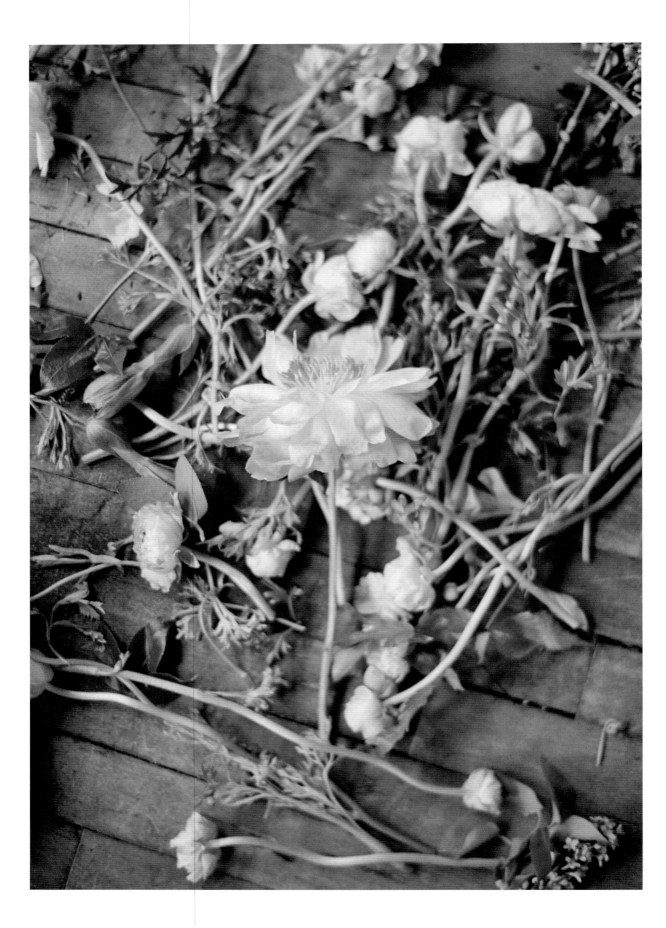

THE FIRST HAIRCUT

My hair started growing back in wispy patches about eight weeks after my last drop of chemo. From the day after the last drop of chemo, each and every morning I ran to the mirror to look for any signs of growth. Most mornings, I was sorely disappointed. As it turned out, I could feel the hair before I could see it.

Speaking of sore, I was surprised by how much the sprouting of my new hair follicles hurt. Yes, hurt. It was the strangest sensation, feeling like an inside-out cactus. Yet when they broke through my scalp, to the touch, they felt like the fur of a baby chick. After a couple of months, I looked like a cross between a Chia Pet and a baby llama. The HOTY and Lalee loved to rub my head, and it felt so good when they did!

There is nothing in the world like the first post-chemo haircut. It took nine long months between my last haircut and this one (well, not counting the head shave!). I can't tell you how happy and excited and even a little nervous I was about it. It felt so odd to be sitting in the same hairdresser's chair after what felt like a lifetime.

Upon my sitting in front of the mirror, my hairdresser told me that I looked especially unusual (yes, she used that word) because each strand of my hair was the same length. Hmm . . . the concept of *each* hair being the same length was simultaneously amusing and perplexing to me. There is no other time in our lives when we literally start from scratch. Literally, every strand of hair starts from ground zero. Even most babies are born with *some* hair.

To add to my unusual appearance, my hairdresser pointed out that the hair on the back of my head was growing in a circle. Yes, a circle. I had Hurricane Chemo on the back of my head. The Silver Lining was that I was grateful for each and every strand.

I've heard many people say that their hair grew back differently: blond became brunette; straight became curly; thin became thick. After the third haircut, mine resembled the same head of hair that I had *before*. The Silver Lining was that I used to wear my hair short before my diagnosis, which meant that I was able to look like my old self in a few months.

> ### LIFELINE
> *Though it varies for everyone, for some people new hair growth can be quite uncomfortable. This is normal & no cause for alarm.*

> ### LIFELINE
> *It can take several weeks or even months for hair to start growing back. You may feel it before you see it.*

BEAUTIFUL, GLORIOUS SLEEP

One of the very frustrating aspects about breast cancer was the insomnia. It started when I had to take pre-chemo steroids. Oh, those were awful days of feeling jittery, anxious, grumpy, *and* sleepless. The only thing that enabled me to sleep was potent pills, but even on medication, it wasn't deep and restful. Prior to beginning them, I talked with my doctors about the drug dependence that I knew would develop.

There is a big difference between drug addiction and drug dependence, though the terms are often mistakenly used interchangeably. Drug addiction is a psychological condition that drives a person to satisfy his or her need for a drug and to keep satisfying it, no matter what. Drug addiction is a compulsive behavior that undermines a person's ability to function. Addiction demands more and more, regardless of the consequences, which can provoke criminal activity resulting in jail time. A person who is addicted to something thinks only about how and when to get the next fix.

LIFELINE

Work closely with your doctors to help wean you off of sleeping pills.

Drug dependence, on the other hand, refers to a state in which the body comes to expect something for normal physiological functioning to occur, such as sleeping pills for sleep. Dependence is the body's adaptation to a substance in such a way that the sudden removal of it will lead to physical withdrawal. Another good example of dependence is a coffee drinker's use of caffeine. If a person is used to drinking several cups of coffee each day, the absence of it often results in a very cranky mood and a headache.

So, over the course of my treatment, I (knowingly) developed a dependence on sleeping pills. But my doctors agreed that it was better for me to get some sleep—even if chemically induced—rather than no sleep at all.

During this recovery period, under the direction and close supervision of my doctors, I weaned myself off of all sleeping medication. Though it was hard and I had to endure several sleepless nights, after about two months I began sleeping on my own, which was a magical Silver Lining.

LIFE'S GREAT METAPHOR

My eight-week recovery from implant surgery coincided with the one-year anniversary of the end of my treatment. The moment that my plastic surgeon gave me the great and glorious news that I finally (!) could start jogging again (albeit slowly), I hopped on a treadmill. I set the speed to 5.5 miles per hour, which was nice and slow for me.

I figured that running on a treadmill was quite like riding a bike . . . hop back on and resume where I left off. I could not have been more *wrong*.

About three minutes into the treadmill run, I lost my balance. First, my right knee went down, then my left. I held on to the railing with my left hand, knees and feet dragging behind. Then—oh, this was the worst part—I tried to get up, while the treadmill was still *moving*. Can you imagine? Trying to stand up on a *moving* treadmill (at jogging pace)? Disaster! What a mess. After about two seconds of calamitously trying to get up, I couldn't hold on any longer and my left hand went down to brace myself and got tangled under my discombobulated feet. Finally, the treadmill sent my whole mangled body shooting off the back end, ripping the headphones from my ears in the process. All of this happened in less than thirty seconds.

Did I mention that I was at a gym? And that it was crowded? There was a wave of gasps, a couple of screeches, and one exceptionally loud f-bomb (from a muscle man lifting weights in the adjoining room). I did the only thing I knew how to do. I got up, brushed myself off, and got back on the treadmill.

As I started jogging again, ridden with scrapes, bruises, and knots and an equally damaged ego, I wondered: "What is the Silver Lining of being spit off the back end of a treadmill?"

I realized instantaneously that this calamitous mishap was analogous to my experience with breast cancer. In the last year, my body, mind, and spirit were mangled by disease. I was physically and emotionally bruised and beaten, just as I was when I was spewed off the treadmill. However, the Silver Lining was that just as I did on the floor of the gym, post–breast cancer I picked myself up, brushed myself off, and got back on the treadmill of life.

The other lesson that I learned was that just as I was unable to resume running on the tread-mill as I had done before, I was unable to resume my life where I left off when I was diagnosed. No, that's not how things work. Things are different now. I am forever changed by breast cancer. I'd like to think for the better. I'll continue to run, both on the treadmill and in life, but just a little more slowly . . . at least for the time being.

> ## LIFELINE
> *Recovery takes time & patience. It cannot be rushed or forced. The more you push, the longer it will take.*

It was during recovery that I had the stark realization that I was now officially a lifetime member of a club to which no one applies and no one wants to join. However, the Silver Lining is that this club has amazingly strong, inspiring, and astounding members. ♥

The *R*s of Recovery

REclaim my life.

REhabilitate my mind, body, and soul.

REnew relationships.

REverse chemo brain, 'roid rage, fatigue, and insomnia.

REflect on this breast cancer experience.

REconvey my gratitude to family, friends, and health care team.

REalize what makes my heart and soul joyful.

REset my circadian rhythm.

REadjust expectations.

REaffirm that I have not lost my mind.

REappraise my priorities.

REallocate my energy.

REengage with the world.

REorganize my day-to-day life.

REbuild my mind and body.

REciprocate the love, attention, and generosity that I received.

REtire my guilt.

The only thing I did not do was REmarry!

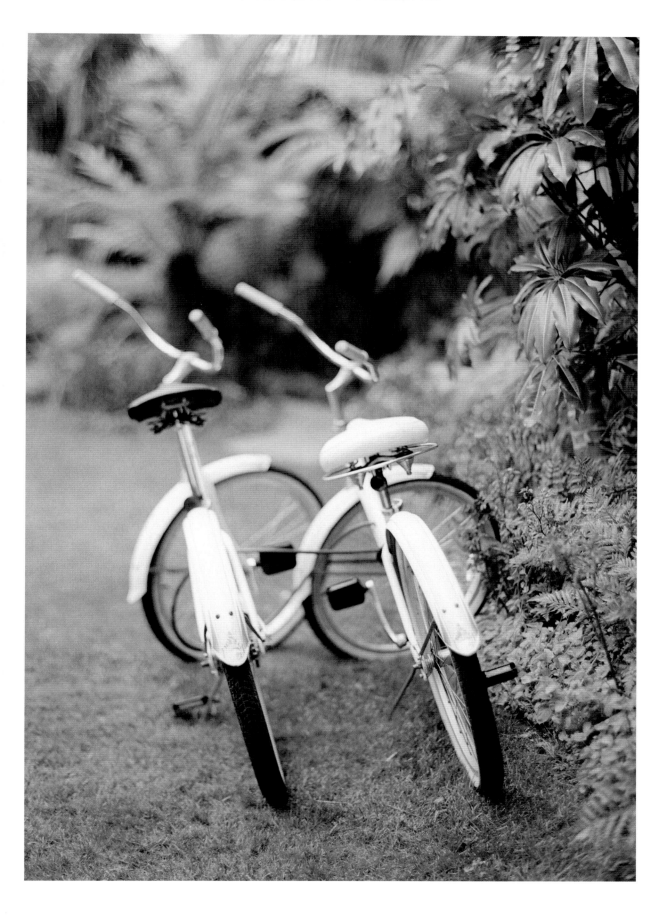

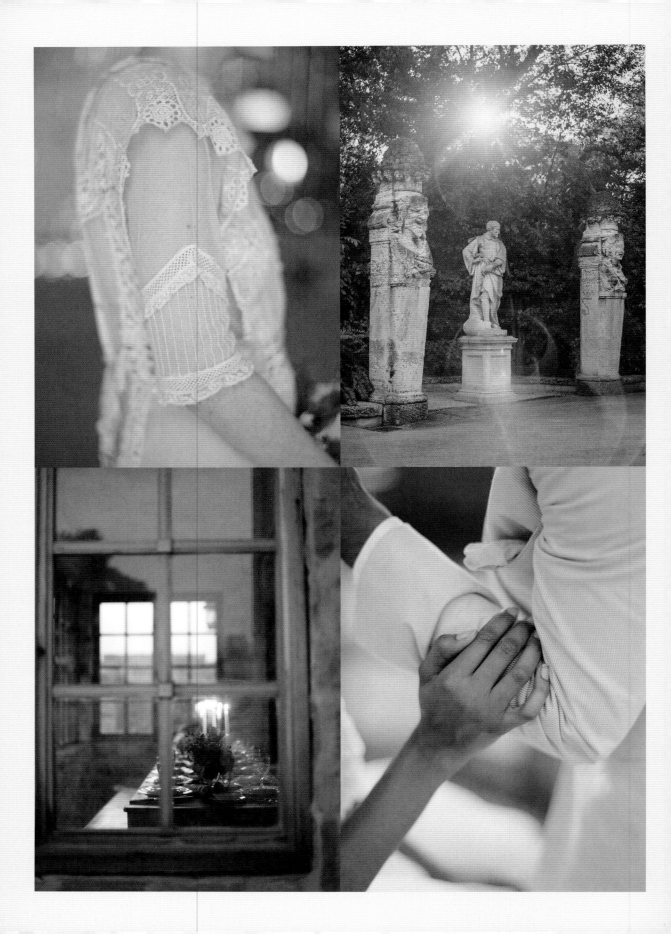

Support & Suggestions

● Make sure that you have a complete, detailed medical record, including cancer diagnosis, every test and the results, surgery hospital notes, all treatments and their side effects, complementary treatments and effects, and clinical trial title and number (if you participated). Be as specific as possible and include dates.

● Grief during and after breast cancer (or any other earth-shattering event) is normal and dynamic, pervasive and individual. I don't think that I have (I *know* that I haven't) fully gone through the grieving process . . . and still have some work to do.

● Returning to your regularly scheduled program is not an option. Like it or not, life is forever changed. Be open to the possibility and Silver Linings that this change can bring.

● Chemo can be pretty devastating to veins, so whenever you have your blood drawn, request a butterfly needle.

● Recovery is the time to decrease or eliminate any drug dependency that you may have developed during treatment, such as on sleeping pills.

● "How are you?" is a very loaded question. Take a deep breath before you answer. Regaining equilibrium in relationships is an ongoing process.

● Making long-term plans becomes feasible after time.

● Honor the feelings and let them out. Prior to my experience with breast cancer, I was a grin-and-bear-it kind of girl who was reluctant to share any feeling other than joy. However, once 'roid rage (the intense feelings of anger brought on by pre-chemotherapy steroids) and Chemo Sobby (tears at the drop of a hat brought on by the chemo drugs) entered my life, I had no choice but to let it all out. And you know what? Expressing feelings, all feelings, happens to feel good. Really good. Though I no longer have either 'roid rage or Chemo Sobby (thank goodness!), I continue to openly express my feelings. And it still feels good!

● Asking for help is a sign of strength, not weakness. It took a cancer diagnosis for me to really get the meaning of this. I now know that seeking support is both the loving and strong thing to do. By getting the right help, whether in making decisions or making meals, I came to realize that letting go of control and delegating is a way to honor yourself and to honor those around you.

● Stop should-ing. Instead of should-ing on myself by guiltily responding to obligation, I now make decisions based on whether it will make my heart sing. That is a great Silver Lining!

● Now is the time to schedule regular check-ups (e.g., dentist, internist, gynecologist) to determine your new baseline.

Questions to Ask Your Oncologist at Follow-Up Appointments

1. How often will I need to see you?
2. What follow-up tests, if any, will I have? When?
3. When do you want me to see my gynecologist? My internist?
4. What symptoms do I need to watch for?
5. What do you want me to do if any occur?
6. What are the long-term or late-onset side effects of treatment? How long will they last?
7. What can I do to prevent the breast cancer from coming back?
8. Can you refer me to someone who can help me on this roller coaster of emotions?
9. What is my survivorship care plan? How will we know if it is working?

Questions to Ask Your Plastic Surgeon Before Implant Surgery

1. What type of implants do you recommend for me? Why?
2. Do you have access to all types of implants?
3. How many breast implant surgeries do you do a year?
4. What is your re-operation rate?
5. How long will the surgery last?
6. What type of pain medicine will I take?
7. What is my expected recovery time?
8. What are the potential complications and how will they be managed?
9. How can I minimize potential complications?
10. How can I tell whether the implants have ruptured?
11. What type of follow-up is required?
12. How long will the implants last?
13. Will my insurance cover this surgery?
14. How will I know if there is a leak? What do I need to do?

How to Sleep Without Prescription Medicine

- Avoid caffeine entirely, but certainly within three to four hours of bedtime.
- Drink herbal tea before bed.
- Turn off all electronic devices (including television) at least one hour before bedtime.
- Avoid stress as much as humanly possible.
- Exercise regularly, ideally five days a week.
- Eat a balanced, healthy diet.
- Avoid alcohol and sugar, especially before bed.
- Sleep in a dark room.
- Read a real hardcover or paperback book or magazine before bed.
- Meditate daily.

Ways to Simplify Your Life

- Evaluate commitments.
- Evaluate time.
- Limit media consumption.
- Spend time with people you love.
- Purge clutter.
- Say N-O.
- Do absolutely nothing ten minutes a day.
- Limit communication.
- Spend time alone.
- Find a creative outlet for self-expression.
- Identify priorities, including self-care, family, friends, and work.

Suggestions to Get Your Sexy Back

- Communicate with your partner.
- Prioritize your sexuality.
- Lubricate.
- Use toys and massage lotion.
- Wax (after the hair grows back)
- Wear sexy lingerie.
- Wear red lipstick.
- Get a manicure and pedicure.
- Keep at it!

Fun Ways to Stimulate Your Brain

- Brush your teeth, eat, or play tennis (!) with your nondominant hand.
- Learn a new language.
- Play an instrument.
- Read a book and answer the book club questions at the back.
- Try new recipes.
- Visit new places.
- Read new authors and genres.
- Do puzzles and brainteasers.
- Memorize a poem.

CHAPTER IX

After

*What Life After Cancer
Treatment Looks Like*

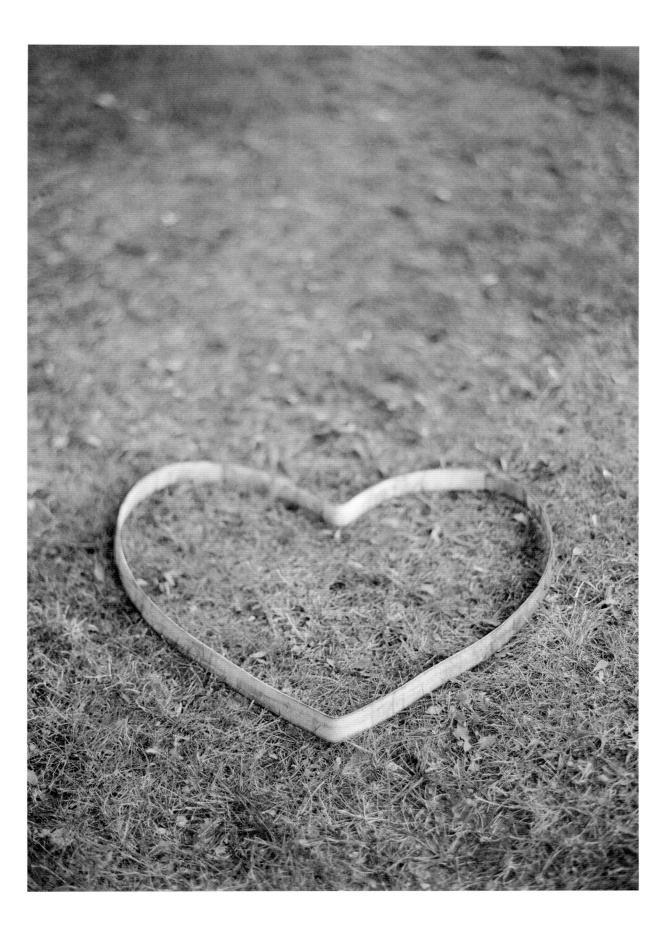

Since finishing breast cancer treatment and recovery, I now find myself in a place of *After*. Life is forever divided between before cancer and after cancer. I am in good company. There are more than 2.9 million breast cancer survivors in the United States today (more than any other group of cancer survivors). Though *After* has a learning curve, it is not nearly as steep and tumultuous as the period between diagnosis and recovery.

My life before breast cancer—as a dinner-making, errand-running, hospice-nursing, carpool-pickup-ing, event-planning wife, mother, friend, and professional—feels like a lifetime ago. However, here I am a mere two years later, happy, healthy, and getting stronger every day. What I have realized is that the experiences of my life prepared me for breast cancer. Though there are still challenges, there is a big, beautiful, and inspiring life beyond breast cancer and this is what it looks like, *After*.

R-ANXIETY

Even though nearly 85 percent of people who have been treated for breast cancer will be cured, because of the unpredictable nature of cancer and the "it happened to me" factor, many people (myself included!) face very real anxiety that breast cancer will come back. Recurrence anxiety is very typical and can, at times, be pervasive. After all, the roots of breast cancer are not only physical but also emotional. The threat of the dreaded *R* is one of the reasons why cancer is such a feared disease. Even long-term survivors continue to experience R-anxiety.

The usual pattern of recurrence anxiety is erratic, with the exception of the immediate period following treatment completion. The first year following the end of treatment is generally associated with the most intense concerns about recurrence.

There are two typical responses to recurrence anxiety: hypochondriasis (suspicion that any physical change or new symptom indicates the cancer's return) and avoidance (whereby physician contact is avoided for fear that physical follow-up could diagnose a malignancy's reappearance). I've definitely had some hypochondria (e.g., Why am I so fatigued? Why does my back hurt? My hot flashes are getting even worse!). I often dreaded seeing

> **LIFELINE**
>
> *Anxiety about a recurrence is a normal part of the healing process. Being present with & processing the emotions are therapeutic ways of coping with the anxiety.*

my oncologist, assuming that today would be the day when the other shoe would drop.

Anxiety about a recurrence is normal. When recurrence anxiety becomes all-consuming, it is important to get professional help so that it doesn't become a debilitating snowball. Begin by talking with your oncologist about it and ask for a referral. I cope by welcoming and addressing my feelings, because if I try to ignore them, they always come back more intensely and often more irrationally. I also remind myself that anticipating things that don't currently exist takes away from life and living. Sometimes when I have a particularly hard time getting off the R-anxiety hamster wheel, I'll go out for a long hike or run. Do whatever you need to do to cope with the very normal feelings that come *after*.

CHANGE

It is typical for people to say that they have changed in one way or another after an experience with breast cancer. Sometimes people are impacted in big ways (e.g., losing weight, smoking cessation, career redirection). Other times, change is more subtle (e.g., taking time to smell the roses). I know without a doubt that I have changed after breast cancer. Though it may sound like a cliché (and maybe it is!), I no longer take my health for granted. My unconscious sense of invincibility is gone, long gone. I am now grateful for what my body can do and respectful of what it needs. I don't push as hard as I used to. When my body says rest, I rest.

I have also started identifying what is really important to me. For example, during this period, I committed to making big and small decisions in my life based on the things that are most meaningful to me, including family, friends, and writing as well as values such as impeccability, curiosity, and flexibility. By knowing what really matters and prioritizing those things, I am able to live a more full and peaceful life.

> **LIFELINE**
>
> *It is valuable to take the time to think about if & how you have changed as a result of breast cancer. Writing is a helpful way to explore these thoughts & feelings.*

What I am (seemingly constantly) reminded of is how little control over earth-rocking events we really have in life. Whether it's a cancer diagnosis or a hurricane, these events will continue to happen. There's no doubt about that. What I do realize, however, is that we *do* have the ability to control how we respond to (inevitable) catastrophe. After breast cancer, I have made the conscious decision to focus on what I can control: my attitude and my perception. If I can't change the stressor directly, then the next best thing is to change my reaction to it. A catastrophe certainly challenges a person's ability to maintain a positive attitude; however, I happen to believe that a

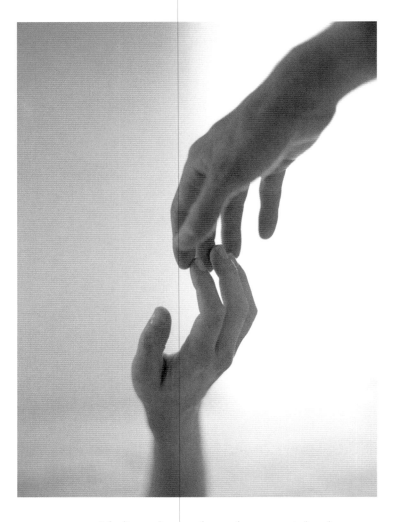

devastating life event can, in fact, bring out the best in a person.

Learning to manage stress has become another priority for me. Stressful things happen in life. The key, again, is how we respond to them. I've learned to cope with stress using restorative yoga, meditation, and even some breathing techniques.

As I moved into the period that I refer to as *After*, another thing that became incredibly important to me was simplifying my life. Truth be told, living simply has never been my thing. I've always had a million balls in the air with omnipresent, complicated logistics.

Instead of rushing from one thing to the next—*hurry-hurry-rush-rush*—I am now drawn to the ordinary. The thought of enjoying a PB&J sandwich (albeit almond butter!) on a blanket in a park is heavenly.

When we simplify our lives, I believe that we have the potential to become more open to other life experiences. A simple life has a different meaning and a different value for every person. For me, it means eliminating all but the essential, eschewing chaos for peace, and spending time doing what's important.

Toward the end of my recovery period, I made a list of things to do to help take the practical steps toward a simplified life. For example, I evaluated my commitments to figure out what I truly valued and loved doing. I eliminated the rest. I also analyzed the time sucks in my life, which led me to limit the time spent tethered to my computer and phone each day. I began spending time only with people whom I love, those folks who energize and enlighten

LIFELINE

Being present with the ordinary in everyday life evokes joy & Silver Linings.

me. I purged my clutter. I learned (and am still learning) to say N-O and eliminate obligation.

Perhaps the most important thing that I did in my quest for a simplified life was to spend time alone, doing nothing. Simplification takes an extraordinary amount of conscious effort; however, it is worth it to acquire more peace, breathing room, space, and focus, which is such a Silver Lining.

As a to-do lister, I get the most benefit from the "task" of sitting in silence with myself. Initially, when I sit in silence, my brain tries (hard!) to fill the space by going in a gazillion different directions at once. The white noise is okay for a short period of time. In fact, I let my brain wander through things for a bit, since this is a good way of determining the specific things I need to let go of. After a few minutes, I ask my brain and my heart to be still and open. I now know the difference between my head and my heart when I observe and listen to both. My brain usually takes me to stressful places, rehashing things I would rather let go of or ruminating on what is to come. My heart, on the other hand, takes me to joy, love, creativity, and Silver Linings.

Stillness is easily found, actually. I find still- ness when I make my morning matcha green tea. Though I'm not a yogi per se, silently doing the child's pose takes me to a peaceful place. Counting the inhalations and exhalations of my breath is another effective way for me to find stillness.

In this *After* period, I have learned to say N-O, though it sure hasn't been easy because I've always been a yes girl with the disease to please. In addition, I have begun to limit my communication. With all the emails, texts, cell phones, and social media, I found myself in digital overdrive. Though limiting my time online hasn't been easy, it has freed a tremendous amount of time that I previously spent looking down. After breast cancer, I'm all about looking *up*.

LINGERING EFFECTS

Breast cancer treatments do, I'm sorry to tell you, have the potential to leave lingering effects. What I know for sure is that breast cancer does nothing slowly or easily.

For example, breasts that have been treated with a lumpectomy or mastectomy can aesthetically look very different from original breasts. I have a whole new chest; every once in a while, when I get a glimpse of myself in the mirror, I gasp and wonder, "Is that *really* me?" The gasp comes from the fact that no matter how good they look under clothes (and they do look good, if I do say so myself!), they are not real breasts. It's still stunning to realize that I am a double amputee.

Scarring can also be troublesome. My post-mastectomy scar is still sensitive and sometimes itchy two years after the surgery. The Silver Lining is that there are lotions that help immensely. Talk with your plastic surgeon about options.

Depending on where radiation is delivered, it can cause scarring and/or hardening of tissues that line the lungs, sometimes resulting in difficulty breathing. The Silver Lining is that there are many treatment options, including steroids for inflammation and inhalers to open airways. Always let your doctor know—immediately!—if you have any of these issues.

Chemotherapy can affect the nervous system, causing numbness and tingling in the hands and feet. After my one dose of Taxol, it took about eight months before I could fully feel my toes. As with all side effects, the timing and intensity varies from person to person.

Long-term studies are now being conducted to investigate the effect of chemo on memory. I know lots of people for whom chemo brain has lingered, myself included. In an effort to proactively offset my lingering chemo brain, I have found that reading, board games, and even sudoku make my noodle work and in turn make me feel a little less spacey and forgetful.

Oh, and then there is the issue of lingering sexual problems, beginning with a low or lack of interest, dryness, and pain, not to mention feeling *un*sexy. When I was on Tamoxifen, the hot flashes added insult to injury. This sexual (non)function has been a ginormous challenge and frustration of mine, not to mention the HOTY's. The Silver Lining is that with time, patience, and commitment, sexuality can be reclaimed. Honest communication with both your doctor and your partner is key. I have spoken with other women who have been in similar circumstances, which has normalized my feelings.

Radiation and chemo can also cause other types of cancers. *GULP!* It's important to pay attention to symptoms, such as a new lump or a thickening in your breast, skin inflammation, a lump or swelling in the lymph nodes under your arm, difficulty breathing, persistent cough, pain, loss of appetite, to name a few. The bottom line is that you know your body better than anyone. Keep a detailed record of these symptoms (including timing,

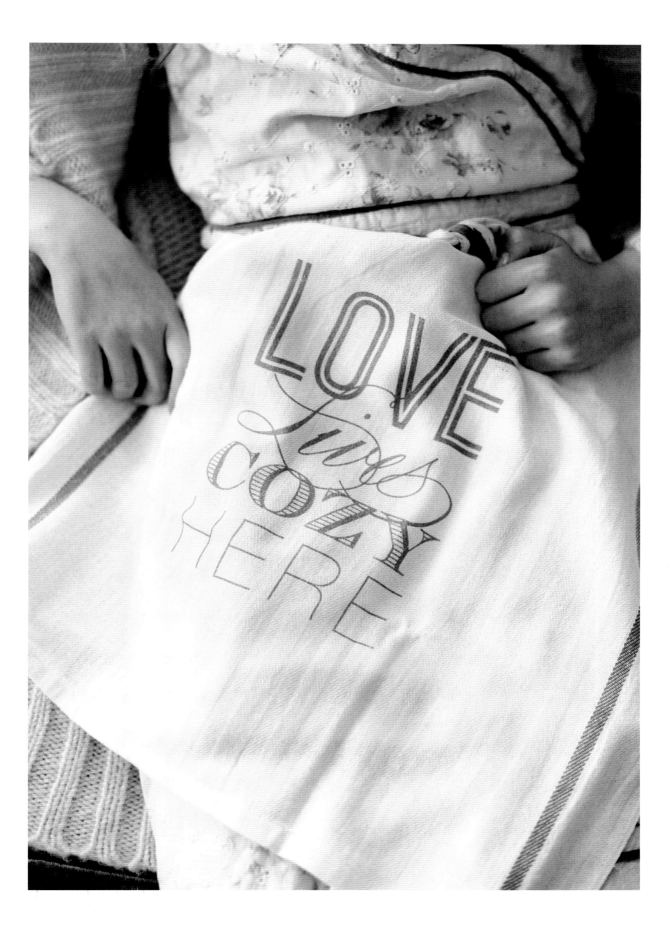

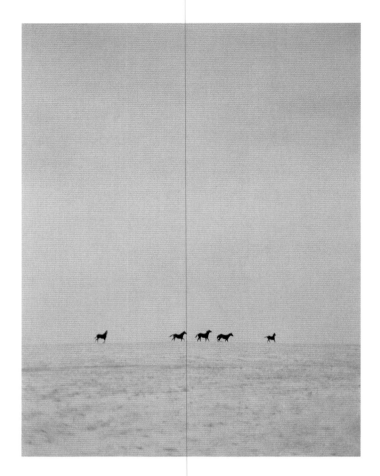

intensity, activity before and after) and be sure to keep your doctor informed.

Fatigue is another lingerer. As Dr. Marisa Weiss points out in her book *Living Well Beyond Breast Cancer,* there are emotional, psychological, and physical causes of fatigue. The uncertainty of a recurrence combined with depression and stress are contributors to fatigue. Additionally, surgery, anesthesia, chemotherapy, and radiation are all very real physical factors that cause fatigue. The Silver Lining is that Dr. Weiss suggests terrific ways to counteract fatigue, beginning with a physical assessment to make sure that there is no medical condition that is causing the fatigue. When that is ruled out, she suggests conserving and allocating energy, getting rest and exercise, consuming the proper fluids and nutrients, and balancing a room's light and darkness.

RISK REDUCTION

From the time of my diagnosis, my sole focus was getting rid of breast cancer. After treatment and recovery, my focus now is on reducing my risk of a recurrence. Though there is not one single way to prevent a recurrence, the Silver Lining is that there are a number of ways that I can take an active role in decreasing the risk that breast cancer would ever come back. Maintaining a healthy weight is at the top of the list.

Studies show that being overweight increases the risk of a recurrence because fat cells produce extra hormones, which is associated with a breast cancer diagnosis. My two favorite ways to keep a healthy weight are exercise and diet. As I have mentioned throughout the book, exercise is very important to me. On average, I exercise six days a week. I'm not saying that to boast. The truth is that if I don't exercise, I get a little stir-crazy and even a tad grumpy.

Exercise has an innumerable amount of Silver Linings, beginning with its ability to decrease and reverse stress. It is a mood enhancer and concentration builder.

Exercise also helps build and maintain healthy bones, which is particularly important *after* breast cancer bone density–depleting treatments.

Studies show that exercise can reduce the risk of a breast cancer recurrence. The NCI (National Cancer Institute) says that "physical activity may prevent tumor development by lowering hormone levels, particularly in premenopausal women; lowering levels of insulin and insulinlike growth factor I (IGF-I); improving the immune response; and assisting with weight maintenance to avoid a high body mass and excess body fat."

The recommendation is to do at least thirty minutes of moderate to vigorous physical activity on five or more days per week. As if that isn't motivation enough to start exercising, an additional Silver Lining of exercise is that the more you do it, the more you want to do it!

Diet is another important factor in maintaining a healthy weight and therefore reducing the risk of a breast cancer recurrence. Though no specific diet can prevent a recurrence, I believe that being as healthy as I can be will help lower my risk of getting the dreaded disease again.

A must-read book on the subject is *Anticancer: A New Way of Life,* by Dr. David Servan-Schreiber. He not only describes the relationship between diet and cancer, but also offers practical suggestions for decreasing the risk of getting cancer. Servan-Schreiber suggests that an anticancer diet needs to be chiefly composed of legumes and vegetables and prepared with flaxseed, canola, olive oil, or omega-3 butter; herbs; and spices. His "Anticancer Plate" includes grains in the form of multigrain bread, whole-grain rice, quinoa, and bulgur; fats in the form of olive, canola, or flaxseed oil and omega-3 butter; herbs and spices such as turmeric, mint, thyme, rosemary, and garlic; vegetables and fruits; and vegetable proteins in the form of lentils, peas, beans, and tofu. He suggests that animal proteins are optional and may be consumed in the form of fish, organic meat, and organic dairy products.

Incorporating the *Anticancer* philosophy and plan into my diet has been very feasible and utterly tasty. My diet has also seen a radical reduction in sugar intake, which has been really hard (as you may recall from my chocolate-malt-guzzling days in chapter seven). Additionally, I have limited my wine consumption because studies have shown that consuming three to four alcoholic drinks or more

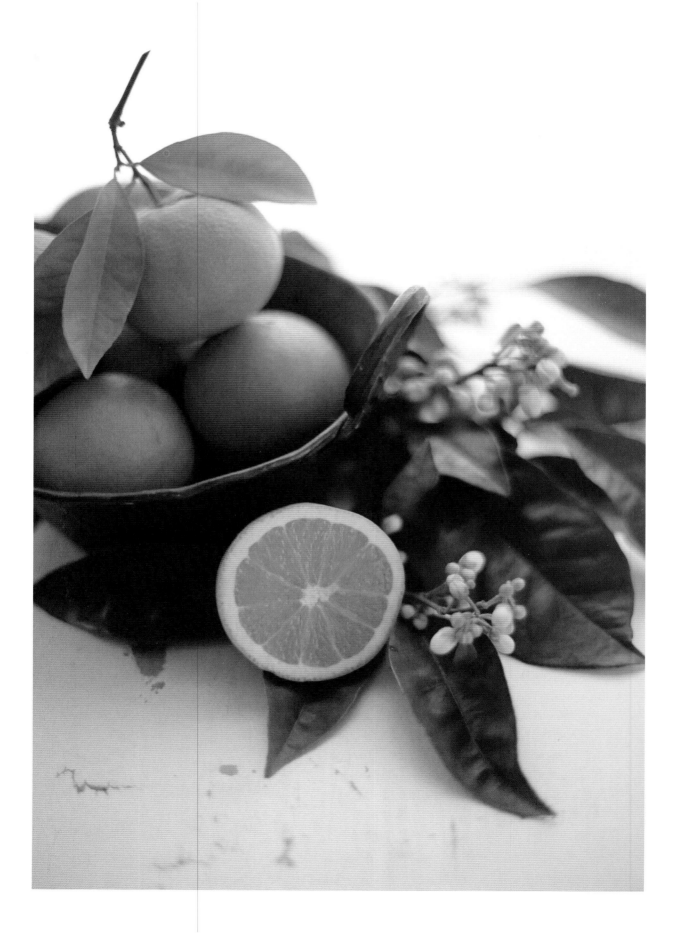

per week after a breast cancer diagnosis may increase the risk of a recurrence. Now, that's not to say that I don't have the occasional ice cream cone or a glass of wine here and there; the key is that I'm much more thoughtful about what I consume and when, which happens to be a Silver Lining.

Another important component of my recurrence risk reduction diet is keeping fat consumption below 20 percent of my total daily calories. When I do consume fat, I make sure that it is the good kind, usually in the form of omega-3 fatty acids. To get my omega-3 fatty acids, I eat salmon twice a week and snack on walnuts. After breast cancer, I have developed a taste for sardines. Don't ask me why. The Silver Lining is that they have lots of omega-3s, twice the calcium content of milk, and are less than two dollars a can!

As you may recall from chapter seven, fiber became my friend and now fiber is one of my best friends. In fact, my goal each day is to get in the neighborhood of twenty-five to thirty grams of it. It may sound like a lot, but it really is doable, especially when you set your mind to it. Vegetables, legumes, and beans combined with a dab of ground flaxseed here and there add up quickly and happily.

I also eat boatloads of cruciferous vegetables, such as Brussels sprouts, broccoli, radishes, arugula, and horseradish, because studies have shown that they help prevent cancer by protecting cells from DNA damage and inactivating carcinogens. Don't you love all of these Silver Linings?

If you saw a dietitian when you were undergoing treatment, it is a super idea to continue the relationship so that you can plan a diet that is geared toward lowering your risk of a recurrence. The Silver Lining is that if you didn't see a dietitian during treatment, it's not too late. Now is as good a time as any to make an appointment! Most cancer centers have dietitians on staff, so it isn't an added cost.

Though I know that there is not one thing to prevent a recurrence, eating a fabulous, nutrient-dense diet and having a strong body will ensure that I am as strong and as healthy as possible to handle whatever comes my way.

When it comes to household products, though there is no official connection between them and breast cancer, there is concern about a variety of products containing hormone disruptors (e.g., parabens and phthalates)—chemicals that when absorbed into the body can mimic or interfere with hormones such as estrogen. Since my breast cancer was ER+, I feel like I have had a lifetime of hormone interference and would prefer to avoid it in the future. Additionally, after having all of the toxicity of treatment, from chemo chemicals to rads of radiation, I'd really

> **LIFELINE**
>
> *Juicing is a deliciously wonderful way to get a whole lot of nutrition in a cup. Many grocery stores now have juice bars. There are also online companies that will ship fresh-pressed juice directly to your front door.*

prefer to stay away from future toxicity as much as possible.

Therefore, in my *After* period, I am committed to avoiding chemicals in my makeup and lotions. For example, I now prefer to use grapeseed oil as my total body lotion. Yep, It's *amazing!* In terms of our household products, we now use only chemical free-cleaning supplies such as lemons and vinegar. They work like a charm! The Silver Linings are that these products are natural, powerful, and—best of all—inexpensive!

GROWING

Two years after my diagnosis, Lalee is doing great, better than great, actually. She is a healthy, well-adjusted first grader who loves *Star Wars* and building sand castles at the beach. Every once in a while, at the most random times, she will ask me about cancer. Last week, Lalee and I had a dialogue that went like this:

"Momma, I never give you leg hugs anymore."

"I loved your leg hugs," I said.

"Would you like one now?" she asked.

"Absolutely!" I said, and she proceeded to hug my legs just in the same way that she did after my double mastectomy. And then, it occurred to her:

"Momma, I've never had a leg hug."

"Would you like one?" I asked.

"Yes!" she said, and then I proceeded to give her sweet little legs a hug.

She has also asked me whether a person can get cancer twice. I am truthful with her and say, "Yes, *but* I'm going to do everything that I can possibly do to prevent it from coming back."

Her response: "I hope it doesn't come back either, but if it does, we will look for Silver Linings."

If we did one thing right during my treatment, it was the way in which we communicated with and included Lalee. Though I wish that this experience had never happened to her, I believe in my heart of hearts that we all did the very best we could. To hear Lalee talk about Silver Linings is one of the greatest Silver Linings I ever could have hoped for.

There isn't a day that goes by when I don't find myself staring at her with thoughts of wonderment and profound joy. Sometimes I go into her room at night to rub her head and listen to her little snore. After breast cancer, every minute with my baby girl is precious.

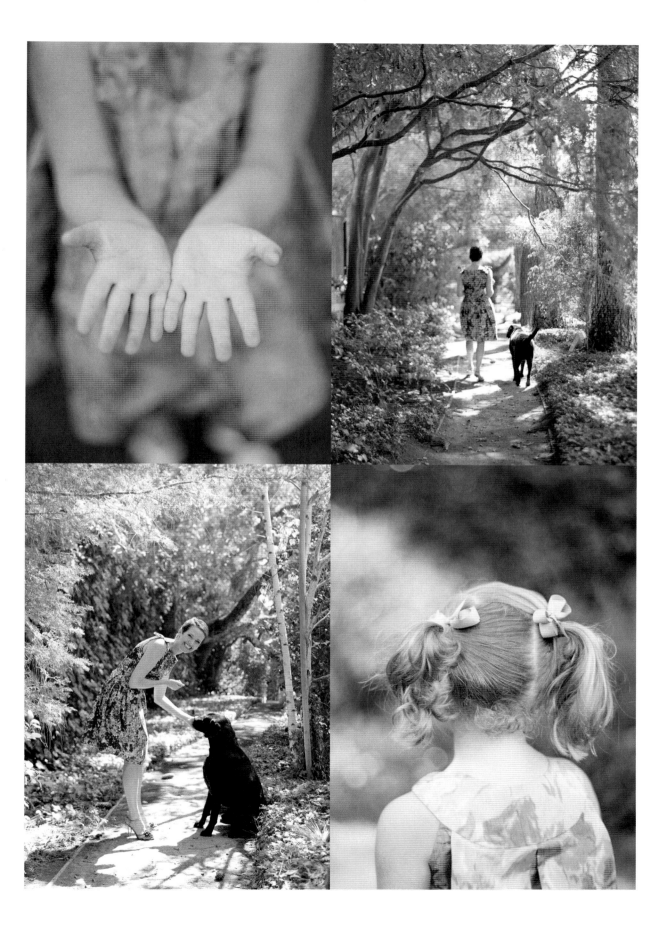

BACK TO WORK

When I started to come out of my dense breast cancer fog, I was eager to reengage with the world. I began with my inner circle of family and friends and gradually expanded to my professional life. By the way, I know how truly blessed I was to be able to take time away from work while I was going through treatment.

As a nurse and social worker, I cared for many patients who were unable to take time off or had to explain every sick day. I vividly remember having to negotiate with employers on my patients' behalf. It's a brutal process. As if having breast cancer isn't bad enough. I mean, really. The two Silver Linings are that (1) I was an anomaly, because many people feel well enough ("enough" being the operative word) to be able to work through treatment, and (2) the majority of employers are understanding and offer supportive flexibility.

As I began to ponder what my professional life would look like, I realized that I had already been "working" every day of my treatment—through the blog. I literally wrote

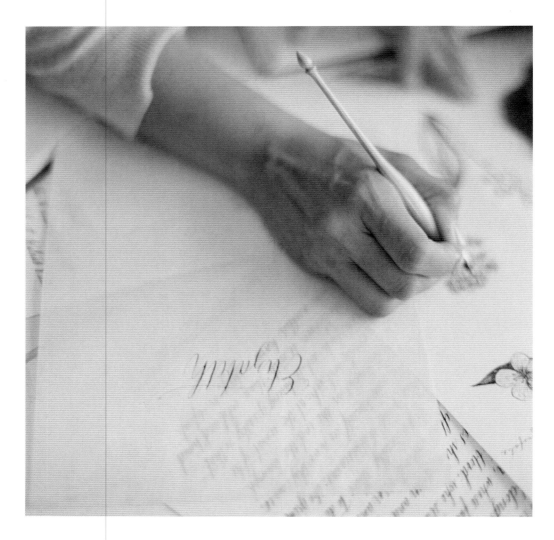

every single day when I was sick. How? you ask. I really don't know, except to say that writing gave me a great deal of pleasure, because I wrote about not only cancer but also travel, fashion, books, children, food, and inspiration. In other words, I forced myself to think and write about other things so that breast cancer was just one part of my life. Yes, there were days (and weeks!) when it was all-consuming; however, giving myself other things to think about was a great Silver Lining.

In terms of my little ol' blog, *The Silver Pen,* I presumed that when treatment was done I would stop writing. Well, it turned out that I still had lots to say, and it also turned out that lots of people still wanted to read. So, I kept writing. And *then,* people started calling me to ask whether I would speak here and yonder. I couldn't have been more surprised. But I took a big courage pill (because speaking about myself was something that I had never done and, quite frankly, terrified me) and said YES!

A wonderfully unanticipated Silver Lining of this whole breast cancer mess is that I now have a new career, as a writer and speaker. I would never, could never have imagined writing the book that you now hold in your hands. Wow. An added Silver Lining is that I went back to clinical work, seeing patients and co-facilitating support groups for children whose parents have cancer. Though I couldn't have imagined it when I was in the bottomless pit of chemo despair, as a result of my experience with breast cancer, my professional life is now more fulfilling than ever before.

AGING

Recently I had the opportunity to attend an incredibly special party. It was so much fun. After breast cancer, I am still so grateful for and enamored of dressing up and going out. It's such a wonderful Silver Lining in my life. During dinner, a friend of a friend (whom I had never met) came over to say hello. She sat down at our table and whined about turning forty. She said, "I just can't believe it. I'm *not* handling aging well." I looked at her and thought, "You've *got* to be kidding? *Really,* lady?"

The day before my fortieth birthday, I had a PORT-A-CATH surgically inserted. On my fortieth birthday, I had a ginormous bandage covering my neck and a tremendous amount of pain from the surgical procedure.

What I know for sure is that I'm really happy—ecstatic, actually—to have the opportunity to have birthdays. I felt sad for this woman who was paralyzed by a number and was unable to celebrate her life, her family, and her health at the beautiful age of forty. Aging is a gift not afforded to everyone. Every year I age is another year that I have lived. This, my friends, is the ultimate Silver Lining. ♥

Being Happy

Being happy means taking a deep breath.

Being happy means doing random acts of kindness.

Being happy means learning something new every day.

Being happy means focusing on acceptance.

Being happy means loving yourself.

Being happy means visiting with a friend.

Being happy means living for today.

Being happy means laughing every day.

Being happy means listening.

Being happy means walking in nature.

Being happy means appreciating more.

Being happy means receiving leg hugs.

Being happy means finding Silver Linings.

Happiness is waiting for you. All you have to do is look for it.

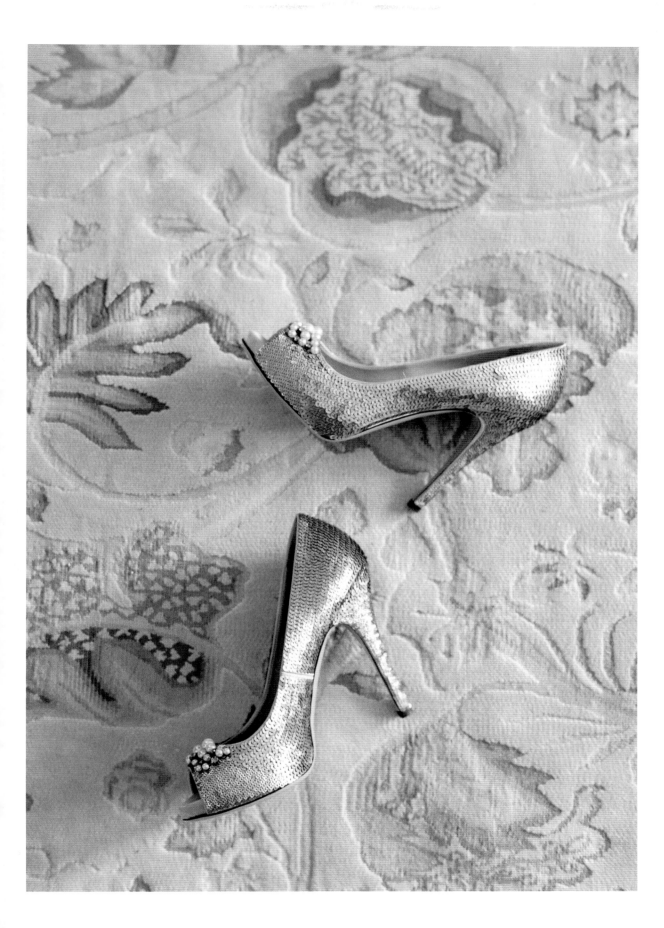

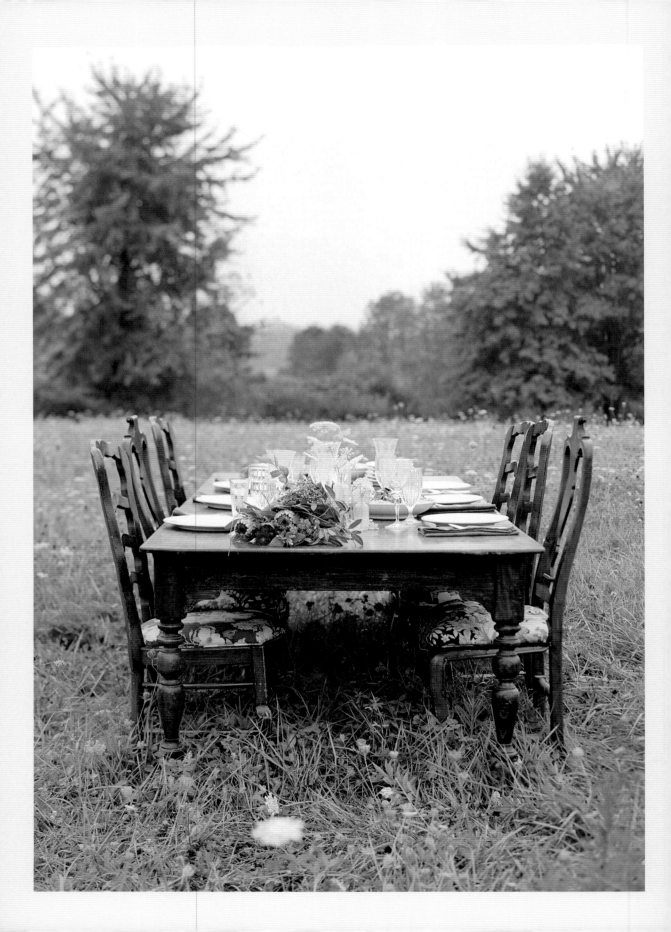

Support & Suggestions

- Recurrence anxiety is typical. If it becomes all-consuming, seek professional support so that it does not become debilitating.
- Take the time to identify what is really important to you and seek fulfillment. After all, if not now, when?
- Maintain a healthy weight. Exercise and diet play a large role in reducing the risk of recurrence.
- Be still and silent for five minutes a day. It will be a gift to yourself.
- Aging is a gift. Celebrate each and every birthday with great love and joy.
- Talk openly with your health care team about lingering side effects.
- Emotionally and physically invest in a survivorship care plan. Partner with your health care team to make it a living and functioning document.

Ways to Maintain a Healthy Weight

EAT HEALTHY, whole grain foods, high-quality proteins, and lots of fruits and vegetables to keep your system working all day and running efficiently. It doesn't have to be expensive. Foods such as brown rice, whole-grain pasta, and frozen vegetables are often less than two dollars per package.

DON'T STARVE YOURSELF. Seriously reducing calories after heavy eating will slow your metabolism.

AVOID SALT and salty foods.

EAT REAL, UNPROCESSED FOOD. Avoid processed foods, especially those with gluten, because they will add to the bloat. Avoid bread, pasta, and crackers and go for salads, vegetables, legumes, and whole grains.

DRINK LOTS OF WATER to help flush the toxins out of your body. Many times when we think we're hungry, we're actually thirsty.

EXERCISE! You don't have to go to a fancy gym. Park at the far end of your work or grocery store parking lot and take the stairs instead of the elevator.

BE PATIENT. Studies show that stress actually leads to weight gain. Successful weight loss takes time. If you feel stressed, take three deep breaths and smile when you do. Repeat as often as necessary to help melt the stress away.

Conclusion

This book is my story. I share this with you because I want to help shed some light on the darkness, to guide you through the confusion, and to hold your hand through the pain. I was trained as a nurse and social worker to heal. When I became a patient, the healing process became personal. I had to learn how to let people care for me, nurture me, and love me when I was at my worst physically, emotionally, mentally, and spiritually. The learning curve was incredibly steep, at times requiring a lifeline, but I did it and so can you.

Are there memories that I would like to forget? Absolutely. Writing this book made me revisit the often excruciating pain of my experience. There were times that my writing gave me a fast pass back to Isolation Island. However, I was buoyed by the inspiring Silver Linings that appeared when I needed them the most.

Life is extraordinary now. I live in the moment, each and every day. After all, this is all any of us really has. Are there hard days? Yes, of course. There are deadlines, fatigue, bills to be paid, traffic, blah, blah, blah. However, now when I am frustrated or sad or confused, I know that consciously stopping myself to look for Silver Linings will ease whatever is troubling me.

Please allow me to acknowledge the special circumstances of the people who are initially diagnosed with late-stage, metastatic breast cancer. I know that your situation is unique and that you face particularly challenging issues. I really, truly, deeply wish that I had the space in this book to address your unique challenges. However, you can always find me on TheSilverPen.com, where I do write about and for you.

What I know for sure is that pain is pain. We are all recovering from something. The pain is hard and the recovery is hard, but if you seek the balance and perspective that Silver Linings offer, you will find them.

I hope that in some small way my experience and my choice to communicate my story will be of help to my fellow travelers and Silver Lining seekers on this tumultuous journey of breast cancer. As I said at the beginning of the book, We. Can. Do. This. There is indeed life—a beautiful, gratitude-filled life—*after* breast cancer. ♥

—Hollye Jacobs

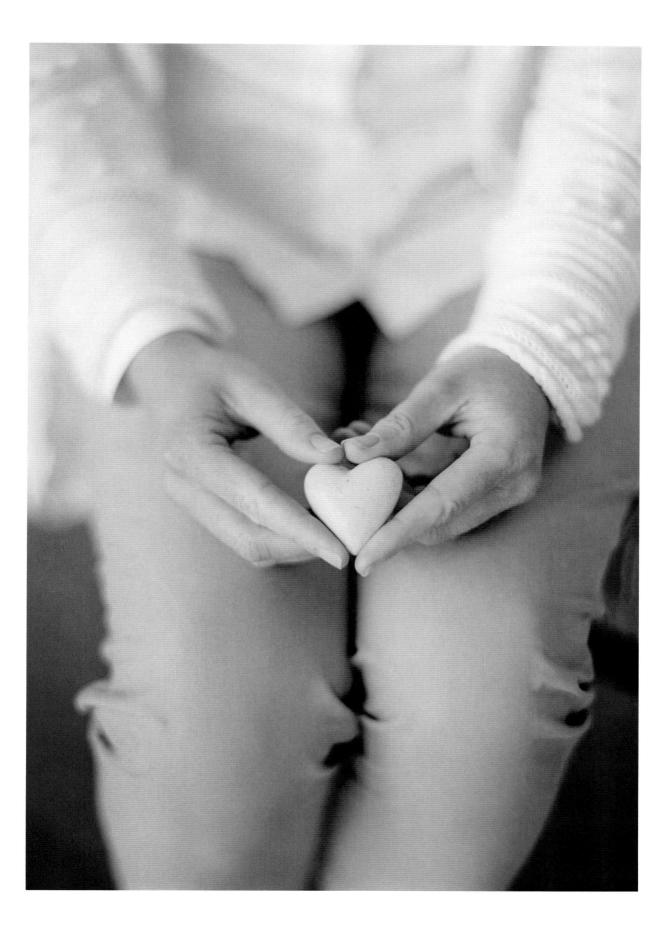

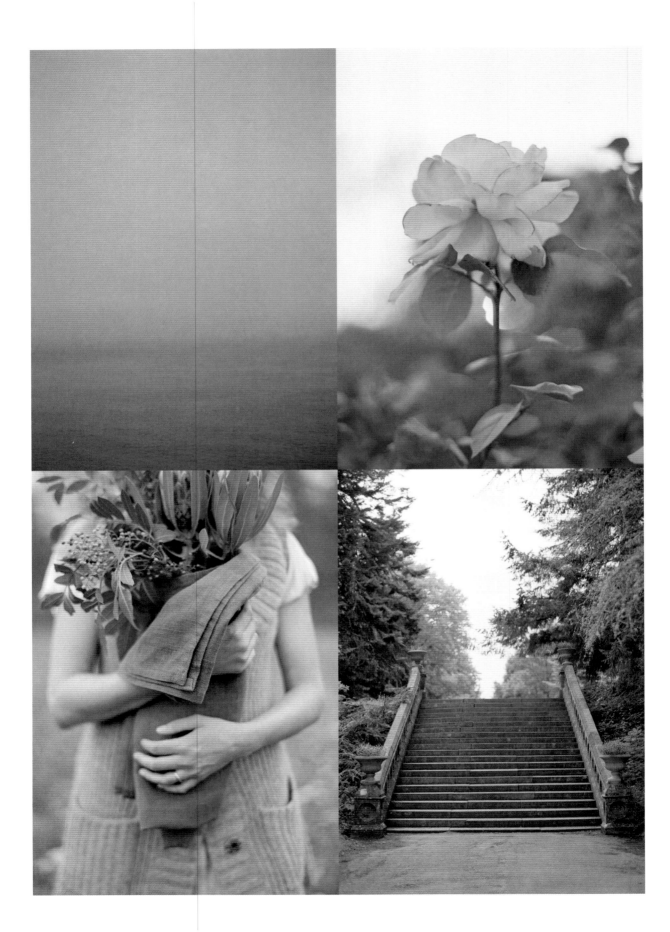

Acknowledgments

It takes a village to go through breast cancer.
It also takes a village to write a book. Neither could
have been done without the unending love and
support of these magnificent Silver Linings:

Kurt Ransohoff, Fred Kass, Marisa Weiss, Michael Kearney, Barbara Fowble, Armando Giuliano, Jay Arthur Jensen, Susan Gibson, Susan Love, Nancy Brinker, Eric Winer, Mark Pegram, Philomena McAndrew, Oprah Winfrey, Lori Thuente, Merryl F. Brown, Marla Phillips, Lisa Wolf, Bernice Kwok-Gabel, Sloan Barnett, Melissa Biggs Bradley, Alexandra Knight, Juliet de Baubigny, Kisa Heyer, Katherine Stewart, Maggie Geyer, Martha Conlin, Doug Turshen, Rebecca Votto, Suzanne Garrett, Deb Peterson, Matt Sanchez, Willow Bay, Marc Chamlin, Debbie Kass, Daryl Stegall, Carolyn Reidy, Judith Curr, Julia Rodgers, Margo Barbakow, David Huang, Marlene Veloz, Sally Jordan, Genevieve Reitman, Mollie Ahlstrand, Radhule Weininger, Jill Cohen, Bob and Robin Fell, Jeff Wattenberg, Robin Cohen, Meika McKrindle, Jackie Gonzalez, Suzy Dobreski, Don and Stacey Fergusson, Yvonne Busch, Kendall Conrad, Carolyn Miller, Gina Tolleson, Howard Bernick, Sarah Branham, Kim Quang, David Schmerler, Clarita Mendoza, Kathy Freston, Sam Silvio, Betty Ferrell, Pam Malloy, Judy Paice, Otis Brawley, Beverlye Hyman Fead, Rhonda Lea Martinez, Adrienne and Haley Carrere, Trish Rooney Alden, Whitney Lasky, Jeff and Amy Mader, Steve and Ginny Simon, Thomas Rollerson, the Dream Foundation, Jeff (HOTY), Ben, Casey, Toby, and Finley Jacobs, Rob Jacobs, Les and Joan Jacobs, Walker Lee Moore, Mykela, Jasmine and Malik Moore, Forum One, Anais Williams, Rich Reisin, Len Friedman, Nancy Koppleman, the entire staff of the Cancer Center of Santa Barbara, and last but not least, Hollye's beloved dog, Buzz, who was by her side every minute of every day.

With love and gratitude,
Hollye & Elizabeth

Glossary

ABSOLUTE NEUTROPHIL COUNT (ANC). Represents the number of neutrophils (a type of white blood cell known for fighting infection) that are present in the blood.

ADJUVANT TREATMENT. Therapy offered in addition to an initial surgical procedure to decrease the risk of relapse. Types of adjuvant care include biological therapy, chemotherapy, hormone therapy, radiation, and targeted therapy.

ALOPECIA. A condition that causes the loss of hair from anywhere on the body, primarily the scalp.

ANALGESIC. Refers to any drug that is administered or prescribed to alleviate pain without the loss of consciousness by blocking the messages transferred between the brain and the pain receptor site.

ANTIEMETIC. Refers to a drug taken to alleviate nausea and vomiting.

APOPTOSIS. The biological sequence of steps whereby certain unwanted cells self-terminate (also referred to as programmed cell death, or PCD), essential to maintaining the body's natural process of cell division.

AREOLA MAMMAE. The circular pigmented area around the nipple of the breast.

AXILLARY (LYMPH NODE) DISSECTION. Refers to the surgical removal of lymph nodes located in the armpit region.

BENIGN TUMOR. A mass of noncancerous cells or tissue that serves no useful purpose and is unable to invade or spread to other parts of the body.

BIOPSY. The removal and microscopic analysis of a small piece of live tissue, performed to determine an accurate diagnosis.

BONE SCAN. A medical procedure that involves a radioactive substance (called a tracer) injected into a vein. The tracer travels from the bloodstream to the bones, allowing for a scanner to photograph the condition of the bones.

BRCA1. A tumor suppressor gene embedded with the instructions to produce a protein that helps maintain healthy cell division and growth as well as repair damaged DNA if possible and destroy if unable to repair. BRCA1 derives its name from being the first discovered hereditary gene mutation associated with a higher risk of developing breast cancer.

BRCA2. A tumor suppressor gene embedded with the instructions to produce a protein that helps maintain healthy cell division and growth as well as repair damaged DNA if possible and destroy if unable to repair. BRCA2 derives its name from being the second discovered hereditary gene mutation associated with a higher risk of developing breast cancer.

BREAST CANCER. The development of malignant (cancerous) cells that originate in the tissues of the breast, usually the ducts and lobules.

BREAST IMPLANT. A prosthetic device consisting of a silicone outer shell and filled with silicone gel or saline (salt water) that is implanted to augment, reconstruct, or create the physical form of female breasts.

CANCER. A term used to describe nearly one hundred diseases characterized by a malignant and invasive tumor caused by the uncontrolled division and growth of abnormal cells.

CANCER CELL. An abnormal cell that divides and reproduces with uncontrolled growth, becoming part of a malignant tumor when combined with other like cells.

CARCINOMA. Refers to any cancer that initially develops in the skin or other tissues, including breast tissue.

CARCINOMA IN SITU (CIS). Refers to a cancer that is present only in the cells where it began and has not invaded or spread to any surrounding tissue.

CATHETER. A medical-grade tube that is either thin and flexible or larger and hard that can be inserted into a body cavity, duct, or vessel to treat diseases or perform a surgical procedure. Catheters may be inserted for temporary use or left in the body permanently.

CAT SCAN (COMPUTED AXIAL TOMOGRAPHY, COMPUTED TOMOGRAPHY, CT SCAN). A cross-sectional image of the body produced by using X-ray technology that may include bone, blood vessels, organs, or soft tissue.

CHEMOTHERAPY. The treatment of cancer that uses chemotherapeutic agents that are selectively destructive and toxic to malignant cells and tissue.

CHRONIC. Used to describe a disease or health condition that has a long duration (more than three months) or recurs frequently.

CLINICAL TRIALS. A biomedical or behavioral research study, or set of tests, conducted on a select sample of human subjects for the purpose of gathering and evaluating data on the efficacy and safety of various diagnostics, devices, drugs, and therapy protocols.

COMPLETE BLOOD COUNT (CBC). A measure of the amount of three types of cells in your blood—red blood cells, white blood cells, and platelets—determined by a cancer blood panel or blood test.

CORE BIOPSY. A diagnostic medical procedure in which a thin, hollow needle is inserted into the lump or mass; the doctor may then obtain a more accurate diagnosis by examining the tissue sample under a microscope.

DUCTAL CARCINOMA IN SITU (DCIS). Refers to a cancer diagnosis where the presence of abnormal cells is discovered inside a milk duct of a breast. It is considered noninvasive, as the cells have not spread to any normal surrounding tissue.

EDEMA. Refers to swelling caused by an abnormal accumulation of excess fluid trapped in the body's tissues.

ESTROGEN. A group of compounds or hormones produced primarily by the ovaries that are responsible for menstrual cyclical changes and for the development and maintenance of secondary sex characteristics.

ESTROGEN RECEPTOR (ER). Refers to a protein receptor found within cells that, once activated by the hormone estrogen, allows the estrogen to bind to DNA, which may cause the cell to grow.

FINE-NEEDLE ASPIRATION (FNA). A diagnostic medical procedure in which a tissue sample is gathered and analyzed for a more accurate diagnosis by inserting a thin, hollow needle (thinner than the needle used for a core biopsy) into a lump or mass that can be felt by hand.

HEMATOMA. A localized collection of blood (usually clotted) outside of a blood vessel, usually due to a damaged artery, capillary, or vein that has allowed blood to leak into tissues where it does not belong.

HER2/NEU (HUMAN EPIDERMAL GROWTH FACTOR RECEPTOR 2). Refers to a gene that is responsible for sending signals to the cells with instructions to divide, grow, or repair. A mutation (HER2 positive) only occurs in certain cancer cells, which promotes the division and growth of the cells; an HER2 mutation is not hereditary. About 15 to 20 percent of all breast cancers are HER2/neu-positive.

HORMONAL THERAPY. A form of systemic therapy, or medical treatment, that uses medications that contain female hormones.

HOTY. Husband of the year.

IN SITU. When the cancer cells are confined or localized to their place of origin and have not spread to the surrounding tissue.

INTERNAL RADIATION (IMPLANT RADIATION, BRACHYTHERAPY). A form of radiation therapy in which the radiation source is within an implant that is temporarily or permanently placed inside the body in the required treatment area. Radiation is slowly released into the body over several months.

INTRAVENOUS (IV). Refers to the administration of a drug, nutrient, or other liquid substance through a syringe or catheter directly into a vein.

INVASIVE CARCINOMA. Refers to cancer cells that penetrate the basement membrane, which allows the cells to invade, or spread, to the surrounding healthy tissue.

LEUKOPENIA. The medical term for a low white blood cell count, which places the body at risk for infection.

LUMPECTOMY. Surgical removal of the breast tumor (the "lump") and some of the normal tissue that surrounds it.

LYMPH. A clear to yellowish watery fluid that circulates throughout the lymphatic system, carrying red blood cells, white blood cells, oxygen, and protein. Lymph also collects and filters out bacteria, fats, and other unwanted material.

LYMPHATIC SYSTEM. Refers to a subset of the circulatory system that consists of lymph ducts, lymph nodes, and lymph vessels, which transport lymph directionally toward the heart. The lymphatic system performs an essential role in maintaining immune health.

LYMPHEDEMA. Refers to localized fluid retention, or swelling (usually in an arm or leg), due to an obstruction in the lymphatic system. Damage to or removal of lymph nodes can cause lymphedema.

LYMPH NODES. Round or oval-shaped structures distributed throughout the body, including the armpit and stomach, that act as filters for harmful substances and contain cells that attack germs and help fight infection.

MAGNETIC RESONANCE IMAGING (MRI, NUCLEAR MAGNETIC RESONANCE IMAGING, NMR IMAGING, NUCLEAR MAGNETIC RESONANCE TOMOGRAPHY). A medical imaging technique that uses powerful magnets and radio waves to produce a high-quality, detailed cross-sectional image of the internal structures of the body.

MALIGNANT TUMOR. A cancerous mass of tissue that has no physiological purpose other than to survive and to grow.

MAMMOGRAM. Refers to a medical procedure that produces an X-ray image of the breast. Mammograms are used by doctors to detect any abnormalities such as tumors.

MARGINS. A term used to describe the visible distance between the tumor that is removed during surgery and the border or edge of the surrounding tissue that is also removed. The margins are microscopically analyzed to determine whether the area is free of cancer cells.

MASTECTOMY. The medical term for the surgical removal of all or part of one or both breasts.

MASTITIS. An inflammation in either one or both mammary glands within the breast that results in redness, pain, and swelling.

MENOPAUSE. The natural biological process during which menstruation and fertility cease, typically defined as occurring the twelve consecutive months following a woman's last menstrual period.

METASTASIS. A complex process that involves the spread of a disease-producing agency from the site of origin to another nonadjacent organ or part.

MYELOSUPPRESSION. Refers to a medical condition, often a side effect of chemotherapy, characterized by a decrease in bone marrow activity that can result in a decrease of red blood cells, white blood cells, and platelets.

NEUTROPHIL. A type of white blood cell that is produced in the bone marrow and circulates in the blood stream. As a type of immune cell, neutrophils are generally the first to respond and arrive at the site of infection.

ONCOGENE. A gene that has the ability to transform a normal cell into a malignant, or cancerous, cell.

ONCOLOGIST. A physician who specializes in the diagnosis, study, and treatment of neoplastic diseases, particularly cancer.

ONCOLOGY. Refers to the study of cancer that consists of three primary disciplines: medical, surgical, and radiation oncology.

OOPHORECTOMY. Refers to the surgical removal of either one ovary, in which a woman may still menstruate and bear children, or both ovaries, which causes a woman's menstruation to cease as well as takes away her ability to have children.

OSTEOPOROSIS. Refers to a disease in which the bones lose density, becoming frail and thin, which increases the risk of fracture.

PALLIATIVE TREATMENT. An area of health care that specializes in relieving and preventing suffering for patients in all stages of serious illness. Using an interdisciplinary approach, this type of care addresses the emotional, physical, social, and spiritual issues of patients and their families.

PALPATION. A form of physical assessment that uses the physical act of feeling or applying light pressure with the hand or fingers to the surface of the body to determine a medical diagnosis.

PATHOLOGY. The scientific study of the nature of diseases, with an emphasis on the structural and functional changes in bodily tissue as a disease progresses.

PROGESTERONE. A hormone made by the body that is important in ovulation, menstruation, and pregnancy.

PROGNOSIS. Refers to a medical opinion assessing the probable course and outcome of a disease, including the patient's estimated chance of recovery.

PROSTHESIS. Refers to an artificial device used to augment or replace an impaired or missing body part.

RADIATION ONCOLOGIST. A physician who specializes in overseeing the use of radiation therapy as a treatment method for patients with cancer.

RADIOLOGIST. A physician who specializes in radiology, or the use of radioactive substances for the diagnosis and treatment of disease.

RADIOTHERAPY (RADIATION THERAPY). The controlled use of high-energy radiation, usually X-rays, as a treatment plan to damage, or destroy, malignant cells by stopping them from dividing properly.

RECONSTRUCTIVE SURGERY. A type of surgery performed to replace the breast tissue and the skin of a breast that was previously removed, with the goal of restoring symmetry between the two breasts.

RECURRENCE. When the disease returns after a period of remission. A local recurrence refers to the disease returning to the site of origin. A regional recurrence refers to the disease returning to the lymph nodes. A distant recurrence refers to the disease returning to parts of the body distant from the site of origin.

RED BLOOD CELL (ERYTHROCYTE). The type of cell in the blood that carries oxygen and carbon dioxide from the lungs to the tissues.

REMISSION. Refers to the period when a disease appears to be inactive. A complete remission indicates no sign of the disease. Partial remission indicates that there is a significant decrease in the number of diseased cells and a few symptoms remain.

SIMULTANEOUS RECONSTRUCTION. The medical term for a surgical procedure that involves both a mastectomy and immediate breast reconstruction.

STAGING. A staging system provides a standardized method for the cancer care team to determine whether the cancer has spread within the breast or to other parts of the body. The breast cancer stage is based on results from the clinical stage, which includes a biopsy, physical exam, and, sometimes, additional blood or imaging tests.

SYSTEMIC THERAPY. Treatment designed to destroy or slow the growth of cancer cells at the primary site, treat cancer that affects the entire body, and attack cancer cells that have spread from the primary site to other organs.

TAMOXIFEN. An antiestrogen commonly used in hormone treatment therapy due to its ability to block the actions of the female hormone estrogen.

THROMBOCYTOPENIA. Refers to any medical condition in which there is an abnormally low number of platelets in the blood, which may result in bruising, bleeding in the tissues, and slow blood clotting after injury.

TISSUE EXPANDER. An inflatable breast implant that is inserted under the skin near the area to be repaired and gradually filled with salt water. The expander is designed to stretch the skin and muscle to create a soft pocket that will eventually contain a permanent implant.

TRAM FLAP. Refers to a surgical procedure that uses the transverse rectus abdominis myocutaneous (TRAM) flap to carry lower abdominal fat, muscle, and skin to the breast in reconstructive surgery as an alternative to a prosthesis.

TWO-STEP PROCEDURE. A medical term that refers to the process whereby surgical biopsy and breast surgery are performed during two separate procedures.

ULTRASOUND EXAMINATION. Refers to a noninvasive, painless imaging method that uses high-frequency sound waves to produce fairly precise images of the body's organs and structures; it is used by doctors to diagnose and treat a variety of medical conditions.

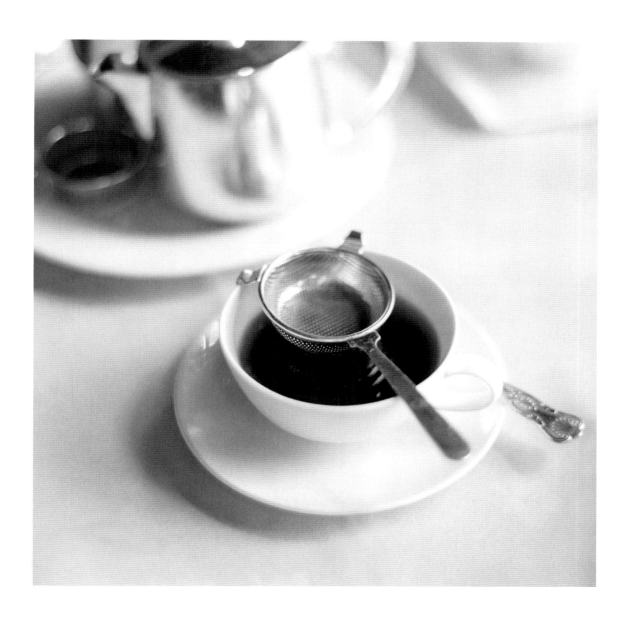

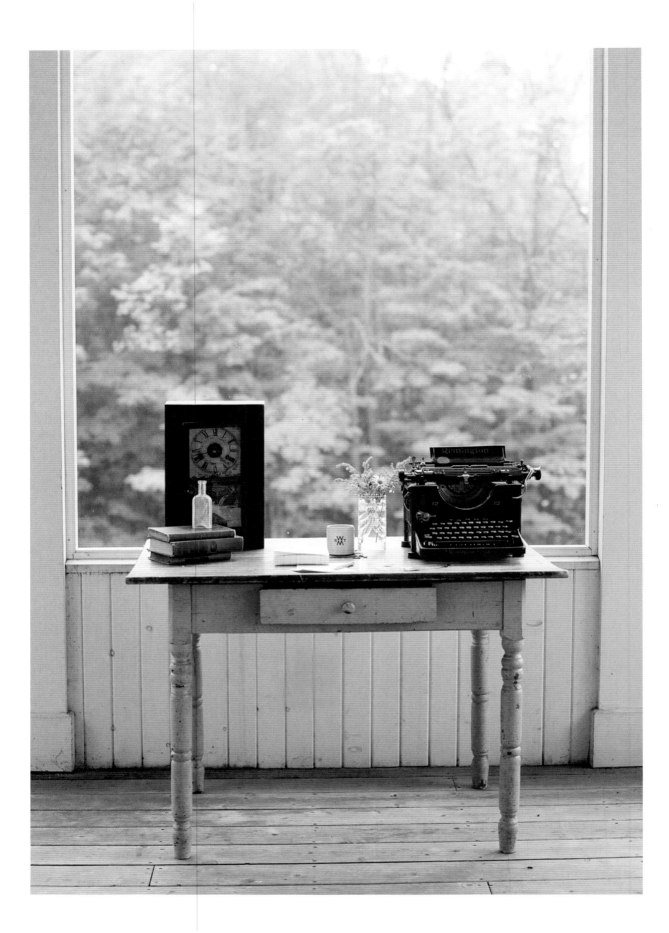

Resource Guide

Academy of Nutrition and Dietetics
www.eatright.org

Adjuvant!
www.adjuvantonline.com

American Cancer Society
www.cancer.org

American College of Radiology
www.acr.org

American Institute for
Cancer Research
www.aicr.org

American Medical Association
www.ama-assn.org

American Psychosocial
Oncology Society
www.apos-society.org/
survivors/helpline/helpline.aspx

American Society of Plastic Surgeons
www.plasticsurgery.org/reconstructive
-procedures/breast-reconstructions

Angel Flight
www.angelflight.com

Army of Women
www.armyofwomen.org

Break Away from Cancer
www.breakawayfromcancer.com

Breastcancer.org

Breast Cancer Freebies
www.breastcancerfreebies.com

CancerCare
www.cancercare.org

Cancer.Net
www.cancer.net

Cancer Support Community
www.cancersupportcommunity.org

Cancer Treatment Centers of America
www.cancercenter.com

CaringBridge
www.caringbridge.org

Dream Foundation
www.dreamfoundation.org

Dr. Susan Love Research Foundation
www.drsusanloveresearchfoundation.com

Fertile Hope
www.fertilehope.org

FORCE (Facing Our
Risk of Cancer Empowered)
www.facingourrisk.org

Foundation for Women's Cancer
www.foundationforwomenscancer.org

Hope for Two: The Pregnant with Cancer
Network
www.pregnantwithcancer.org

Imerman Angels
www.imermanangels.org

Inflammatory Breast Cancer (IBC)
Research Foundation
www.ibcresearch.org

Livestrong Foundation
www.livestrong.org

Living Beyond Breast Cancer
www.lbbc.org

Locks of Love
www.locksoflove.org

Look Good Feel Better
www.lookgoodfeelbetter.org

MD Anderson Cancer Center
www.mdanderson.org

Medscape
www.medscape.com

Metastatic Breast Cancer Network
(MBCN)
www.mbcn.org

National Breast Cancer Coalition
www.breastcancerdeadline2020.org

National Cancer Institute
www.cancer.gov

National Center for Complementary
and Alternative Medicine (NCCAM)
www.nccam.nih.gov

National Coalition for Cancer
Survivorship (NCCS)
www.canceradvocacy.org

National Comprehensive Cancer
Network
www.nccn.com

National Hospice and Palliative Care
Organization
www.nhpco.org

National Institutes of Health
www.nih.gov

National Lymphedema Network
(NLN)
www.lymphnet.org

National Society of Genetic Counselors
www.nsgc.org

NCI-Designated Cancer Centers
www.cancer.gov/researchandfunding
/extramural/cancercenters/find-a-cancer
-center

Office of Cancer Complementary and
Alternative Medicine (OCCAM)
www.cam.cancer.gov

Prevent Cancer Foundation Co-Pay Relief
www.preventcancer.org

Reach to Recovery Program
www.cancer.org/treatment
/supportprogramsservices/reach-to-recovery

Sisters Network, Inc.
www.sistersnetworkinc.org

Stand Up To Cancer (SU2C)
www.standup2cancer.org

Susan G. Komen Breast Cancer Foundation
ww5.komen.org

Triple Negative Breast Cancer (TNBC)
Foundation, Inc.
www.tnbcfoundation.org

U.S. Food and Drug Administration
www.fda.gov

Young Survival Coalition
www.youngsurvival.org

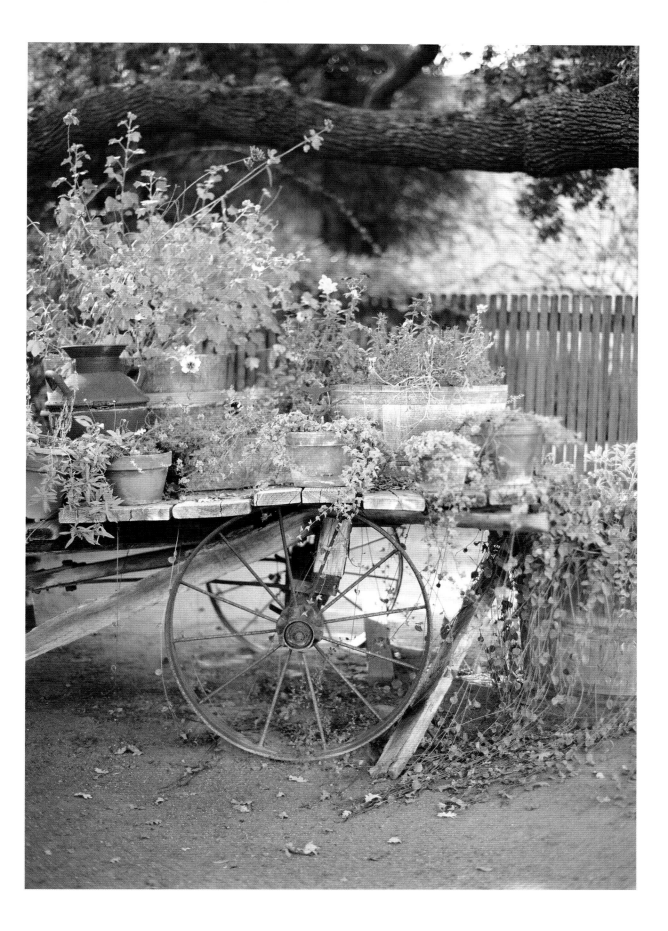

RECOMMENDED BOOKS

ADULT BOOKS

Anticancer: A New Way of Life, by David Servan-Schreiber, MD

Breast Cancer, M. D. Anderson Cancer Care Series, by Kelly K. Hunt, Geoffrey L. Robb, Eric A. Strom, and Naoto T. Ueno

The Breast Cancer Checklist: The Only Guide for What to Do Before, During and After BreastCancer Surgery, Chemotherapy, and Radiation, by Fern Reiss

Breast Cancer Husband: How to Help Your Wife (and Yourself) Through Diagnosis, Treatment, and Beyond, by Marc Silver

Breast Cancer, Real Questions, Real Answers, by David Chan, MD

Cancer: 50 Essential Things to Do, by Greg Anderson

Cancer Vixen, by Marisa Acocella Marchetto

Choices in Breast Cancer Treatment, edited by Kenneth D. Miller

Crazy Sexy Cancer Tips, by Kris Carr

Diagnosis: Breast Cancer, by Cara Novy-Bennewitz

Dr. Susan Love's Breast Book, by Susan M. Love, MD, MBA, with Karen Lindsey

Eat to Lose, Eat to Win, by Rachel Beller, MS, RD

Help Me Live: 20 Things People with Cancer Want You to Know, by Lori Hope

How to Be a Friend to a Friend Who's Sick, by Letty Cottin Pogrebin

Living Well Beyond Breast Cancer, by Marisa Weiss and Ellen Weiss

The Mayo Clinic Breast Cancer Book, edited by Lynn C. Hartmann, MD, and Charles L. Loprinzi, MD

Omnivore's Dilemma, by Michael Pollan

100 Questions & Answers About Breast Cancer Sensuality, Sexuality, and Intimacy, by Michael L. Krychman, MD, Susan Kellogg Spadt, PhD, CRNP, and Sandra Finestone, PsyD

7 Minutes! How to Get the Most from Your Doctor Visit, by Marisa C. Weiss, MD

Taking Care of Your "Girls": A Breast Health Guide for Girls, Teens, and In-Betweens by Marisa C. Weiss and Isabel Friedman

The 10 Best Questions for Surviving Breast Cancer: The Script You Need to Take Control of Your Health, by Dede Bonner and Marisa C. Weiss

What Helped Get Me Through: Cancer Survivors Share Wisdom and Hope edited by Julie K. Silver, MD

FAMILY BOOKS

Barklay and Eve: What IS Cancer, Anyway?, written and illustrated by Karen L. Carney

Child Development: A Practitioner's Guide, by Douglas Davies

How to Help Children Through a Parent's Serious Illness, by Kathleen McCue, MA, LSW, CCLS

Let My Colors Out, by Courtney Filigenzi, illustrated by Shennen Bersani

Nowhere Hair, by Sue Glader, illustrated by Edith Buenen

Our Mom Has Cancer, by Abigail and Adrienne Ackermann

Someone I Love Is Sick: Helping Very Young Children Cope with Cancer in the Family, by Kathleen McCue, MA, LSW, CCLS, illustrated by Jenny Campbell

When a Parent Has Cancer: A Guide to Caring for Your Children, by Wendy Schlessel Harpham, MD

When Mommy Had a Mastectomy, by Nancy Reuben Greenfield, illustrated by Ralph Butler

When Someone You Love Has Cancer: A Guide to Help Kids Cope, written by Alaric Lewis, illustrated by R. W. Alley

RECOMMENDED SHOPPING SITES

Astra Pharmaceuticals
EMLA (numbing cream)
www.astrazeneca.com

BFFL Co. (Best Friends for Life)
The ultimate in friend-to-friend care bags
bfflco.com

Breast Cancer Freebies
breastcancerfreebies.com

Claire Pettibone Lingerie
www.clairepettibone.com

Gebauer Company
Pain Ease (numbing spray)
www.gebauer.com

Headcovers Unlimited
www.headcovers.com

Healing Threads
Kimono-type hospital gowns
www.healingthreads.com

Heavenly Hats
heavenlyhats.com

Mastectomyshop.com
www.mastectomyshop.com

Only Hearts Inner Outerwear
www2.onlyhearts.com

Walker Valentine Custom House
Amazingly soft pajamas, nighties, robes, and handkerchiefs
www.walkervalentine.com

About the Authors

HOLLYE JACOBS, RN, MS, MSW

Hollye Jacobs is a nurse, social worker, child development specialist, speaker, and author. Diagnosed with breast cancer in 2010, she speaks publicly and writes about her experience on the award-winning blog *The Silver Pen* (www.TheSilverPen.com).

She worked as an adult and pediatric palliative care nurse, social worker, and educator for more than fifteen years at the University of Chicago Children's Hospital, the City of Hope medical center, the University of Chicago Pritzker School of Medicine, and Northwestern Memorial Hospital.

Hollye's professional knowledge as a health practitioner and her personal experiences as a cancer patient and survivor present a powerful package. People benefit from her insights, humor, and informed perspective on the breast cancer cycle—from detection to treatment to recovery. Hollye is the experienced girlfriend who tells you what to expect, holds your hand, and helps you find the Silver Linings during the breast cancer experience.

In addition to writing *The Silver Pen,* Hollye also contributes to *The Huffington Post*, Breastcancer .org, Susan G. Komen, and the Dr. Susan Love Research Foundation Army of Women blog.

ELIZABETH MESSINA

Elizabeth Messina is world-renowned photographer. Her artful images grace the covers and pages of countless magazines. She is also the author of the award-winning blog *Kiss the Groom* (www.kissthegroom.com).

Elizabeth has beautifully photographed many celebrities, including Brooke Shields, Lisa Ling, Kevin Garnett, Tiffani Thiessen, and many more. The intimate moments she documented of her dear friend Hollye Jacobs, which fill the pages of this book, are among the most meaningful images she has ever captured.

Elizabeth earned a BFA with honors from the San Francisco Art Institute. Elizabeth is sought after for her masterful use of natural light and film. She was named one of the "Top 10 Wedding Photographers 2008" by *American Photo* and won the 2012 Award for Best Film Portrait Photographer.

Elizabeth's first book, *The Luminous Portrait,* was published in 2012. In it she shares her secrets to creating lush and poignant images. She's also a regular contributor to *The Huffington Post* and has a devoted following of admirers on Instagram (@elizabethmessina).

When she is not creating photographs, you'll find Elizabeth happily nestled in her Southern California home with her Silver Linings: her husband and their three beautiful children.

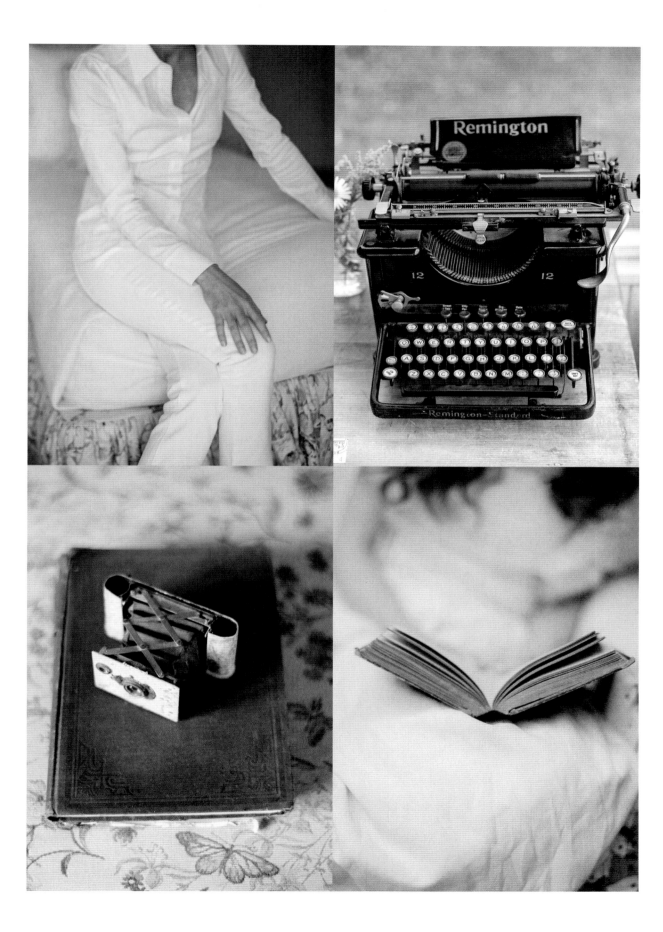

Index

hugs, 49–50, 88, 236

humor, therapeutic effect of, 26, 141, 186–87, 190

hydration, 132

hypochondriasis, 226

I

imagery, 193

immune system, 136, 172, 176, 177, 192

implant reconstruction, 91, 222

implants, 48, 70, 82, 201
    displacement of, 202–3
    semipermanent types of, 200

infections, 132

infiltrating ductal carcinoma, 19, 36

inflammation, 105, 164, 183, 230

inflammatory breast cancer (IFC), 36

inhalers, 230

inner resources, 137

in situ (IS), 35, 250

insomnia, 120, 124, 137, 183, 187, 199, 210, 216

inspiration, 180

insurance, 67, 72, 74, 90, 108, 132, 172

integrative medicine, *see* complementary therapies

internal mammary lymph nodes, 33

internal radiation (implant radiation
    brachytherapy), 250

internet:
    food shopping on, 177
    inaccurate information on, 60
    support systems on, 142

internist, 221

interviewing doctors, 156

intravenous fluids (iv), 76, 78, 102, 104, 105, 110,
    116, 136, 250

intuition, instincts, 6, 11, 26, 67
    of children, 40–41, 54–55

invasive carcinoma, 32–34, 98, 250

invasive ductal carcinoma (IDC), 19, 35, 36

invasive lobular carcinoma, (ILC), 36

isolation, feelings of, 136, 140, 142, 145, 147, 172, 197,
    207, 213, 244

itchiness, 115, 203, 230

J

jogging, 216–17

journal, importance of, 13, 90, 101, 132, 151, 227

joy, 236, 239, 243, 244

JP drains (Jackson-Pratt drains), 82–83, 84, 92, 93

juicing, 235

K

kindness, 143

knitting, needlepoint, 187

K-Y Liquid, 212

L

labels, 176, 236

"lady lumps," 83, 88, 100

languages, 223

language skills, 138, 140

latissimus dorsi flap, 91

laughter as medicine, 186–87, 190

Leader Dogs for the Blind, 185

"leg hug," 49–50, 236

legumes, 233, 235

leukopenia, 250

libido, 124, 199, 210, 230

Lidocaine, 16, 112–13

limits, of body, 227

lingerie, 223

listening skills, 146

Living Well Beyond Breast Cancer (Weiss), 232

lobular cancer in situ (LCIS; lobular neoplasia), 36

loss, feelings of, 196–97

lotion, 235
    for massage, 223
    for radiated skin, 162
    before radiation, 168
    for scar tissue, 230

love, 185–86, 229, 240, 244

lubrication, 212, 223

lumpectomy, 20, 155, 156, 229, 250

lump in breast, 35–36, 230

lymphatic system, 37, 98, 154, 193, 250

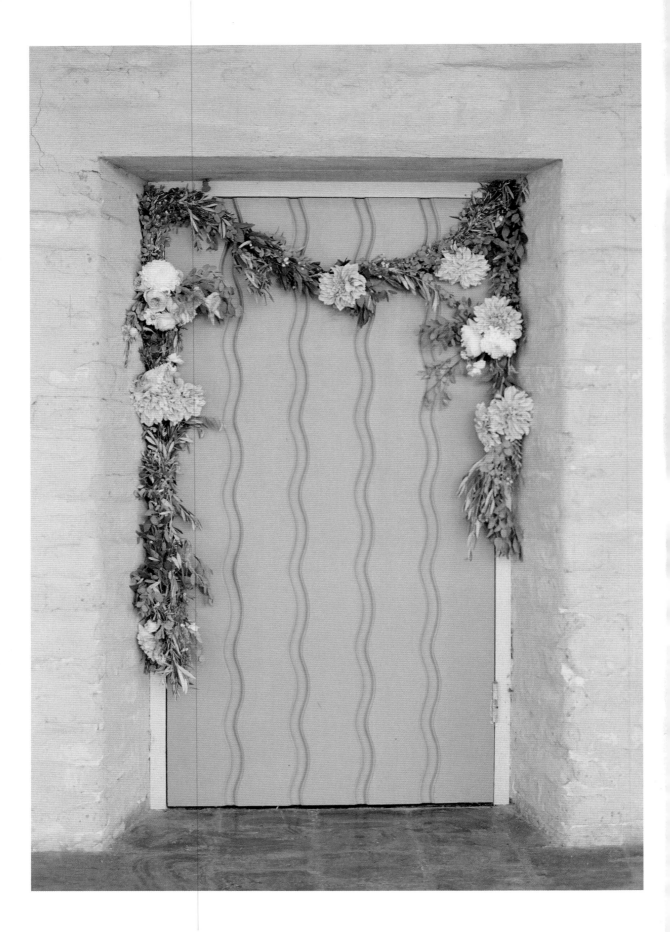